FOREWORD REVIEWS
ForeWord Clarion Review
Health & Fitness

When Cancer Hits Home
***** (5 stars out of 5)

Although discussions about cancer have come a long way since the days when the word was whispered, if even said at all, there's still a need for clear, straightforward information on the topic, believes Dr. Patrick Maguire, author and cancer specialist. Providing treatment options for common cancer types as well as prevention advice, Maguire offers a well-written and much-needed guidebook that will be appreciated by anyone affected by this challenging diagnosis.

Maguire was inspired to write after the loss of both his parents and his father-in-law to cancer within a short time frame. As an oncologist, he'd had abundant exposure to the workings of cancer, but his personal experience helped him to add a different viewpoint: that of a family member watching a loved one go through treatment and loss. These two perspectives, of knowledgeable physician and of family caretaker, combine nicely to give chapters a blend of research and warmth.

In the book's first part, Maguire focuses on cancer prevention, looking at the latest recommendations for reducing cancer risk. Starting with the relationship between cancer risk and nutrition, Maguire digs into dietary data, but admits that many questions remain, and he expresses frustration at the "snake oil salesmen" who prey upon people's fears and hopes with so-called "cancer prevention" foods and products. Even with that caveat, his information is hugely useful and backed by numerous research studies.

Exercise also plays a vital role in reducing cancer risk, he notes. Citing extensive research on the topic, particularly for breast cancer and lung cancer, Maguire adeptly makes his case for why everyone should spend less time on the couch and more time on the move.

For those facing a cancer diagnosis themselves, or dealing with friends or family who are undergoing treatment, the book's second section-on common cancer types-should prove invaluable. Maguire covers the twenty most common types, including breast cancer, leukemia, liver cancer, melanoma, ovarian cancer, and colon cancer. He starts each section with a patient's story, created from the thousands of real patients he's met and treated during his years as an oncologist.

With a friendly tone that helps boost the understanding of complex material, Maguire presents important terminology without bogging down his explanations with medical jargon. Key concepts for each cancer type are included, as well as warning signs and symptoms, staging process and treatment options.

Maguire's talents as a writer are likely the same as his skills as a physician: he articulates risks, research, and treatment in a straightforward, informed manner, but also includes thoughtful, personal stories that connect him to patients and their experience. Whether someone is looking for cancer prevention tips or trying to learn more about a specific cancer, this guide should prove to be a stellar resource.

Elizabeth Millard
ForeWord Reviews

Cancer Survivors & Experts Praise *When Cancer Hits Home*:

"An excellent resource for cancer patients, their families, and medical professionals. The section on breast cancer gives an up-to-date and well-written analysis of the highly complex process of diagnosis and treatment of this disease in a way that is useful and easy to understand."
  - Pamela Garmon, Medical Physicist and Breast Cancer Survivor

"Everything that Dr. Maguire has written in the chapters on prostate cancer and PSA examinations rings true to me."
  - Arnold Palmer, Professional Golfer and Prostate Cancer Survivor

"The read was easy and clear to understand even for non-doctor types...After reading through the percentages, I blew them out of the water (six years and still ticking)! My words of wisdom to patients are to wear the cancer fight like your favorite pair of jeans and get on with life!"
  - Ralph Petite, Husband, Dad, and Melanoma Survivor

"As a breast cancer survivor of 7.5 years, I can tell you that everything Dr. Maguire has written in *When Cancer Hits Home* on breast cancer screening and treatment options is absolutely true."
  - Ollie Burton, Banker and Breast Cancer Survivor

"Without a doubt, what Dr. Maguire discusses in When Cancer Hits Home about PSA screening and prostate cancer treatment is true. I'm a prostate cancer survivor of 2 years."
  - Willie Burton (Ollie's husband), Retired, Prostate Cancer Survivor

"After reading the chapter on uterine cancer (endometrial cancer) in When Cancer Hits Home, I couldn't help but relate my own story to this well written description of the signs and symptoms. I am sure this book will be of great value to those who have battled or know of someone battling this disease."
  - Sue Pasquarell, Administrator, Endometrial Cancer Survivor

"Very well done. The clinical stories are excellent."
 - Christopher Willett MD, Professor and Chair, Department of Radiation Oncology, Duke University Medical Center

"Dr. Maguire has presented the most common urologic malignancies in a very concise and understandable manner. This book will be a great resource for patients and families who are afflicted with and trying to understand their disease and treatment options."
 - Michael Hoffman MD, Urology Clinics of Winchester, Virginia

"*When Cancer Hits Home* provides critical information to patients and their loved ones about treatment options for liver cancer and pancreatic cancer. The author does so in a manner that's down to earth and easy to understand. I think readers will find the personal stories very helpful."
 - John Martinie MD, FACS, Hepatobiliary Surgeon, Carolinas Medical Center

"Outstanding explanation and summary for patients, families, and many of the medical professionals involved with cancer patient treatment...helpful for patients to prepare for initial consultations as well as to reflect upon during treatment. Dr. Maguire has provided a unique, honest, and compassionate way to introduce these discussions."
 - Charles Dye MD, Associate Professor of Medicine, Division of Gastroenterology, Foregut Cancer Group, Penn State College of Medicine

"Patients with lung cancer face difficult and complex problems, and the choices regarding therapy may be difficult to understand. This monograph provides a clear and succinct summary of lung cancer and its treatment options, which will provide a better understanding of this disease and will improve decision making."
 - Thomas A. D'Amico MD, Professor of Surgery, Chief of Thoracic Surgery, Duke University Medical Center

When CANCER Hits HOME

Cancer Treatment and Prevention Options for Breast, Colon, Lung, Prostate and Other Common Types

PATRICK MAGUIRE, MD

DISCLAIMER

This book is not intended to take the place of personal medical advice or to provide medical instruction. All medical advice and counsel must be obtained directly from a physician or other appropriate healthcare professional. Readers who fail to consult with the appropriate healthcare provider assume all risk of injury.

The purpose of this book is to serve as an educational tool for the reader to learn and enhance their knowledge about common cancers in non-medical terms. The information provided herein is believed to be accurate as of the date of publication. The opinions expressed herein are based on the professional judgment and experience of the author. There is no guarantee that the reader will have the same experiences or outcomes discussed in the book.

THIS BOOK IS PROVIDED BY THE AUTHOR ON AN "AS IS" BASIS, AND ANY EXPRESS OR IMPLIED WARRANTIES, INCLUDING, BUT NOT LIMITED TO, THE IMPLIED WARRANTIES OF MERCHANTABILITY AND FITNESS FOR A PARTICULAR PURPOSE ARE DISCLAIMED. IN NO EVENT SHALL THE AUTHOR BE LIABLE FOR ANY DIRECT, INDIRECT, INCIDENTAL, SPECIAL, EXEMPLARY, OR CONSEQUENTIAL DAMAGES HOWEVER CAUSED AND ON ANY THEORY OF LIABILITY ARISING IN ANY WAY OUT OF THE USE OF THIS BOOK, EVEN IF AUTHOR IS ADVISED OF THE POSSIBILITY OF SUCH DAMAGE.

No part of this book may be copied, modified, or used in any way without the express written permission of the author.

Author photo on back cover by Nigel Bibler

ND: 4846-2310-8615, v. 1

DEDICATED...

To Barb, Dave, George, and Sandy

THANK YOU...

To Jill, Julia, Liam, my extended family and friends
for the love and memories that sustain me.

To my colleagues in the medical, radiation,
and surgical specialties for their expert advice.

To the patients, doctors, and staff of Coastal Carolina
Radiation Oncology and New Hanover Regional Medical Center
for teaching me more than I could ever hope to teach them.

TABLE OF CONTENTS

WHEN CANCER HITS HOME

I've been thinking about George today. He would've been 76. That's not too bad: 76. He lived his life hard but honest (well, mostly!) and enjoyed it. George always treated me like his own son. I couldn't have asked for a better father-in-law. He died six years ago from prostate cancer that had spread throughout his blood and his bones. George was one of those guys who never went to the doctor. He started to have a difficult time urinating, so much so that he almost couldn't pee at all. He made a quick trip to the emergency room. The prostate specific antigen (PSA) level in his blood was 250. Normal PSA level for most men is less than 4. Two years later, he was gone.

Wish I could say that was our only loss. George's ex, Sandy, my mother-in-law, was a classy lady. I sometimes kidded with my wife that if her mom was our age, I would've married her instead. She was attractive, street smart, charming, and always looked sharp. Sandy lived for her grandchildren! After we moved from Philly to Carolina, she'd visit frequently and stay with the kids so Jill and I could get out together for a nice dinner or a couple of cocktails. She'd made this most recent trip down to help with our daughter's "Welcome to Preschool" party. Sandy had been telling Jill about this nagging pain in her back. It'd been going on for a couple of months, but clearly was getting worse. I walked in our front door with the newspaper that Sunday morning and saw her sitting on the couch in the living room. She was sobbing, and this was not a woman who cried easily. Her pain had gotten unbearable. We were off to the hospital. A few hours later, the radiologist was showing me the MRI images of her spine. "This can't be anything but cancer," he said. She was dead in six weeks!

Well, at least we still had my parents! They were both retired, my dad from a commercial HVAC company, where he was the purchasing agent, and my mom from the railroad, where she was an administrative assistant. Although they were enjoying their leisurely years, both were plenty tired of shoveling snow and scraping ice every winter in Bucks County, Pennsylvania. They had no problems when I suggested that they move south, especially since they'd been aching to be closer to their grandkids anyway.

All was good for awhile, until my dad started to get extremely tired…all the time. Dave could spin a yarn a mile long about distant relatives, sports stars from the 1950s, bad movies that nobody had ever seen but him, even a classic 20-minute impromptu speech during an Eagles game one year about how to make a good Philly hoagie. My college buddies still laugh about that one! When he got too tired to tell his tales, I knew something wasn't right. He failed to mention the couple of episodes of dark bowel movements that he'd been having. It didn't take his doctors long to find the source of his problems, a large stomach ulcer. He needed an operation, and he got it quickly from a very skilled surgeon. What we weren't expecting was the cancer in the ulcer.

Barb was the one I expected to leave us first. My mom had smoked two to three packs a day from birth. At least it seemed that way to me. I almost couldn't picture her without a smoke and a romance novel in her hands. Much as I loved her, I found it tough to fathom how she could put a cigarette between her teeth even before she brushed them in the morning. But then, that's addiction, I guess?!

One morning before work, I stopped at my parents' house so that I could drive my dad to his doctor's appointment. It'd been a couple of months since his surgery. His doctors needed to run a light down into his stomach to make sure that the cancer hadn't returned. He greeted me at the door with a confused look. Since he'd lost so much blood from the ulcer, then took another hit from the surgery to remove it, his mind hadn't quite recovered. It was like he was in a constant fog. The upbeat, talkative guy that I knew all of my life was gone, and this new guy had taken his place, still very sweet, but much too quiet. That particular morning, however, something else was wrong. As soon as I walked in the front door, I heard the alarm buzzer from my parents' bedroom. My dad said "Mom won't open the door, Pat." I checked myself.

The door was actually unlocked, which I hadn't expected. There she was, lying on her side, hands under her head, peaceful, almost like she was still sleeping...but clearly not. It was the week before Christmas, 2006. When I called my aunts and uncles (and there are many in our large Irish family on both sides), they were anticipating bad news about my dad. That sad day was to come just three months later.

Thinking about it all again today keeps it as raw as I can stand. I know cancer. I've dealt with plenty of it in my first 42 years, thank you very little. Now I'd like to be done with it. Only one problem: I'm an oncologist.

Why Did I Write?

Cancer isn't a topic that most folks look forward to reading about. Unfortunately, it's one that many people find themselves needing to read about. Cancer kills nearly 600,000 people per year in the United States, very similar to the number of deaths caused by heart disease. Virtually everyone knows someone, a relative, a friend, a co-worker, who's been diagnosed with cancer. Breast, colorectal, lung, and prostate cancer, "the big four," together are diagnosed in about 750,000 people per year in the United States alone. Fortunately, our society has come a long way from the days when "She's got the cancer" was whispered quietly at dinner parties and family gatherings. However, a shocking number of myths and misconceptions still thrive.

As a doctor who sees and treats dozens of patients with cancer every day, I've been asked countless questions about it. Some of these questions are specific to the treatments that are being recommended, side effects, and chances for cure. Other inquisitive patients and family members ask, "What is cancer? What could I have done to prevent it? How could I have found this earlier?" These are all excellent questions that prompted my writing.

You'd think, with nearly limitless information at most people's fingertips, that there's not much need for a book to cover these topics. At least, that's what I assumed initially. However, I've found as both a provider and a consumer of cancer care services for my family, that's just not the case. Unfortunately, there are countless Web sites and books in print about cancer treatment or prevention that are so misleading as to be potentially harmful. There are a few excellent resources that aim to guide patients through treatments for specific cancers. Dr. Susan Love's book about breast cancer and Dr. Patrick Walsh's book about prostate cancer are fine examples. There are multiple textbooks to guide oncologists (cancer specialists) and other medical professionals in their care of patients. Personally, I've also been inspired reading several patients' stories of their own journeys. There aren't, however, many good books to educate people about cancer in language that's easily understood. My intent with writing this book was to fill that niche by creating a commonsense guide to common cancers.

While I consider myself a good doctor, I'm neither the smartest nor the most well-known oncologist in America. My promise to myself and to my patients is that I continually strive to improve. It's a work in constant progress. However, if I do have a gift in my relationship with patients and their families, it's the ability to describe the complex and often scary process of cancer diagnosis and treatment in plain terms that are clear and easy to understand. Fear of the unknown weighs heavy. If I'm able to lessen that fear with this book for even a few people, then I'll have achieved my goal.

Who Should Read This?

The short answer to that question is anyone who wants or needs to learn more about cancer in plain, commonsense language. Specifically, you may benefit from reading this book if you:

- want to reduce your risk of being diagnosed with cancer;

- want to learn more about how cancers can be diagnosed at the earliest stages and, therefore, provide the best chance for cure;

- have been recently diagnosed with cancer yourself, or someone close to you has been diagnosed, and you need to know about cancer treatment options, risks and benefits.

As opposed to many other books or Web sites that contain information for the public about cancer treatment or prevention, this guide is based on scientific evidence, described in simple terms. Whether it's risk reduction, early diagnosis, or treatment of individual cancer types, each chapter includes most of the major medical studies that cancer specialists and other doctors use to support their decisions in helping patients. In fact, general medical professionals (primary care physicians, nurses, medical students, and residents) may find the guide to be of assistance in their care of patients who wish to reduce their risk of cancer or are struggling with understanding the process of diagnosis, the stages of cancer, and treatment options.

Format and Recommendations

Part I, "Reduce Your Cancer Risk," is written for anyone who wants to minimize his or her chances of a cancer diagnosis. The main sections of Part I discuss recommendations for the most prevalent cancer-causing agents to avoid, active choices about nutrition and lifestyle changes to consider, as well as specific cancer screening tests to undergo in order to maximize the chance for early diagnosis. These sections could be read individually or all at once, the latter likely in a day or two at most. Whether or not you know someone with cancer, there are major potential health benefits to be gained by learning the concepts and guidelines in Part I.

Part II, "Cancer Treatment Options for the 20 Most Common Types," is written specifically for patients with cancer and those who care for them, both physically and emotionally. Medical jargon is minimal throughout the book to ensure ease of understanding. However, the most important cancer-related terminology is defined for further reference in "Essentials of Cancer Diagnosis, Staging, and Treatment," the first chapter in Part II. Each subsequent chapter is devoted to a specific common cancer site or type, with personalized patient stories at the beginning and end. These stories are based on a compilation of the thousands of real patients that I've met and/or treated over the past 14 years as a cancer specialist. Their purpose is to highlight key concepts about each cancer type. After the beginning of the patient story through diagnosis, each chapter proceeds with a general overview of that particular type of cancer. Included are warning signs and symptoms of cancer, red flags that may signal its presence. A summary of the diagnosis and cancer staging process follows. Current cancer treatment options (as of this writing in 2010) are then discussed in detail. Each chapter concludes with the treatment and outcome for the fictional patient in the story. Not all of the stories have happy endings, unfortunately, just like in real life.

The chapters are listed alphabetically by disease site for convenient reference. Readers will likely want to first delve deeply into those chapters that are most acutely pertinent to their lives. Other chapters can be read later, to improve general knowledge about cancer diagnosis and treatment. Since many types of cancer are very common, unfortunately most people will have more than one type affect their family and friends during their lifetime.

That said, there will undoubtedly be people who read this guide and become acutely concerned that they or someone close to them has cancer. Whether it's a nagging symptom or a new lump, questions and anxiety may arise. There is no substitute for a thorough discussion and physical examination with your primary doctor. Absolutely nothing within this book should take the place of that important relationship.

What is Cancer?

Most people have no reason to think about cancer unless/until they're directly affected by it. Unfortunately, since it's an exceedingly common disease, that time comes for almost every family in the United States. At that point, many people will ask the basic question, "What is cancer anyway?" There are entire textbooks dedicated to the underlying mechanisms of cancer development and progression. However, the best definitions are often the simplest. In order to understand cancer, one needs to understand the cancer cell. The key characteristics of a cancer cell that make it different from most normal cells in the body are its abilities to grow unregulated by the body's defense, the immune system, and usually (though not always) to metastasize or spread to distant sites in the body through lymphatic channels and blood vessels. Cancer cells arise generally from damaged DNA, the building material that makes cells. Some people are born with this damaged DNA, thanks to their parents. Inherited cancers constitute about 10% of all cases in the United States. For most other patients who develop cancer, however, most of the damage occurs as a result of exposures or events that occur after they're born.

In an ideal world, cancer wouldn't exist. Although that's not yet the case in the real world in 2010, we're fortunate to have thousands of brilliant scientific minds working toward the goal of eliminating cancer. Until we achieve that ultimate goal, our short-term goals need to be focused on reducing the numbers of patients who are diagnosed with cancer and, for those who have a cancer diagnosis, to increase their chances for cure. Part I of this guide is largely dedicated to the former goal, while Part II is aimed at the latter.

PART I

REDUCE YOUR
CANCER RISK

AVOID MAJOR MISTAKES

One of the greatest gifts that my dad passed on to me was his attitude of worrying only about the things that were within his power to change. When it comes to cancer, people can't change their genetics (at least not in 2010). On the other hand, they can change certain other aspects of their lives that affect their risk of a cancer diagnosis or death. As with virtually any self-improvement goal in life, reducing cancer risk involves mindfulness and some difficult choices. People who are willing to make those decisions and take positive action will tend to live longer, healthier lives than those who aren't.

To paraphrase the legendary billionaire investor Warren Buffett, the number one rule for investing is, "Don't lose money!" This sounds intuitive and simple, yet it's astounding the number of people who fail to follow this advice when possible. It does actually take money to make money, since you can't grow what you don't have. The first major rule of cancer risk reduction is similar to Mr. Buffett's rule on investing: avoid major mistakes. As with investing, hundreds of thousands of people miss this major point and put themselves dead center in the crosshairs for a future cancer diagnosis. Carcinogens (cancer-causing agents) must be avoided. The list of known or probable cancer-causing agents is extensive. For those interested in an exhaustive review on the subject, the "Report on Carcinogens, Eleventh Edition," from the U.S. Department of Health and Human Services, is a reasonable choice. However, the majority of common cancers that are caused by exposure to a known carcinogen are limited to a select few offenders. These main culprits are the focus of this chapter.

Tobacco Products

If given the opportunity to remove only one product from the planet, totally and forever, most cancer specialists would choose cigarettes. Of those cancers that are linked to a clear source, more are related to smoking cigarettes than any other. Virtually everyone knows that cigarette smoking causes the vast majority of lung cancers. Roughly 90% are estimated to be due to smoking. However, the risks for developing many other types of cancer are significantly increased by smoking. It's been known for several decades that cancers of the lips, mouth, throat, lungs, esophagus, bladder, and even the female cervix are clearly linked in many cases to cigarette smoking. In addition, a cause-and-effect relationship has been shown for cancers of the sinuses, stomach, kidneys, and liver. Fifty years ago, about 40% of adults smoked cigarettes. Over that time span, roughly 14 million people died prematurely as a direct result of cigarette smoking. Without a doubt, the single most important decision that a person can make to minimize the risk of a cancer diagnosis is to avoid using or quit using tobacco products, especially cigarettes.

Viruses

Among the multitude of viruses in the world, only a few have been clearly shown to commonly cause cancer. These include the human papilloma virus (HPV), the hepatitis B virus (HBV), and hepatitis C virus (HCV). The human immunodeficiency virus (HIV) that causes AIDS places patients at increased risk for several types of cancer. Lastly, the Epstein-Barr virus (EBV) appears to play a role in predisposing patients to a couple of types of common cancers.

HPV has long been known to cause the sexually transmitted disease known as genital warts. However, infections with certain strains of HPV also place women at increased risk of cervical cancer. Thanks to widespread use of the Pap test over the past several decades, advanced cervical cancer is much less common in this country, although it remains prevalent worldwide. HPV infection is the main source of cervical cancer. While many women will be infected with HPV, most women's immune systems will eventually clear the virus from their body. These women won't develop cervical cancer.

Unfortunately, other women will be unable to clear the HPV infection, and a proportion will go on to develop invasive and potentially deadly cervical cancer. Over the past few years, however, vaccines against these most virulent strains of HPV have been developed. They are now recommended for girls and young women ages 9 to 26 in order to prevent cervical cancer. Many patients who develop cancer of the anus will have HPV as a source also. It seems likely that vaccination may prevent a large number of these cancers in both sexes.

Interestingly, these same strains of HPV have been linked to a subset of patients with cancer of the throat, particularly in an area of the body called the oropharynx. Doctors began to notice that certain patients who didn't have the usual risk factors for developing throat cancer, namely long-term tobacco or alcohol use, were developing cancers of the oropharynx. Further study of these patients and their tumors revealed evidence of local infection with the most virulent strains of HPV. Discussion is now being held about potentially expanding recommendations for the vaccines against HPV to include boys. Vaccinating boys and young men against these most aggressive strains of HPV will decrease risks to unvaccinated young women and will hopefully decrease the boys' risks of developing squamous cell cancers (those that arise from the superficial lining) of the throat, particularly for those that also don't smoke.

There are three main types of viral hepatitis (liver infection): A, B, and C. Hepatitis A isn't known to increase the risk for any type of cancer. On the other hand, HBV and HCV are both passed from person to person through blood or sexual contact most often, and both can increase the risk of hepatocellular carcinoma (HCC, liver cancer). HBV usually causes flulike symptoms and sometimes jaundice (yellow skin and/or eyes), but most people recover from the acute illness. The small subgroup that goes on to become chronic carriers of the virus is at higher risk for developing liver cancer. Fortunately, a vaccine is available to prevent HBV. While most people are able to get the vaccine, it is most commonly offered to children and groups of adults who are at high risk for infection, such as health care workers. HCV is less likely to cause symptoms than HBV. In fact, the majority of people who are infected actually don't know it. Those who have chronic HCV are at increased risk for liver cancer. Unfortunately, there's no current vaccine for HCV. Although the vast majority won't develop cancer of the liver, they're at significantly increased risk compared to the general population.

HIV, the virus that causes AIDS, isn't known to directly cause any type of cancer. However, it's thought that by suppressing the body's immune system, HIV prevents repair of damaged cells, some of which may progress to become cancer cells. These common types include lymphomas of both Hodgkin and non-Hodgkin types, lung cancers, liver cancers, and squamous cell cancers of the cervix, anus, and skin. Over the past two decades, highly active anti-retroviral therapy for AIDS has transformed the disease into a chronic illness for those that are able to obtain the medications. In addition to the rare Kaposi's sarcoma (depicted on Tom Hanks's face in the movie *Philadelphia*), non-Hodgkin lymphomas have become less common thanks to these effective medicines. However, other cancers remain very common in patients with AIDS, including an apparently increasing rate of anal squamous cell carcinomas, particularly among gay men.

EBV, the virus that causes mononucleosis, is prevalent in the United States and in the world. It's well known that this virus is spread by sharing saliva, coughing, sneezing, etc. The vast majority of those infected have no major health problems as a result, and the virus remains dormant in a type of immune cell in the body. However, EBV has been linked to a couple of common cancers. People who are infected with EBV have an increased risk of cancer of the nasopharynx (the area behind the nose, in front of the brain), a type of head and neck cancer. There's also a suggested relationship between EBV and Hodgkin lymphoma. Lastly, the virus has a clear link to the development of Burkitt's lymphoma, although this subtype is rare.

Medical Treatments

Ironically, the same treatments that are used to treat cancer can also have a small risk of causing cancer in the same patient years later. Chemotherapy, anti-cancer medications usually given by vein or by mouth, has a slight risk of causing cancer in patients who receive certain medications. The class of chemotherapy drugs classically associated with subsequent risk of cancer induction (starting) is alkylating agents. Many of these drugs are no longer widely in use, since effective, safer alternatives have taken their place. While the chance of developing a cancer after chemotherapy overall is less than 1%, the most common type that occurs in this setting is a type of leukemia called acute myelogenous (AML).

Radiation therapy (RT) also can cause cancer. While the few patients that develop treatment-related cancers after chemotherapy usually have them occur within a few years, second cancers caused by RT may not arise until a decade or more later. As opposed to chemotherapy alkylating agents that classically may cause AML, RT most commonly may cause secondary solid tumors. Second tumors caused by RT are rare in absolute terms, also occurring in much less than 1% of patients treated. However, the risk and type of cancer development after RT depends on multiple factors, including age of the patient, body site treated, and RT dose delivered. In general, children are much more susceptible to developing RT-induced cancers than adults. Larger treatment areas and higher RT doses may increase the relative risk.

Nature

"All natural" is not always "all good." Strictly in terms of numbers, non-melanoma skin cancer is by far the most common cancer in the United States. Tens of thousands of people visit dermatologists and surgeons each year for removal of these skin cancers. While there may be a genetic component that can't be changed, the vast majority of these cancers are due to excessive sun exposure. Mother Nature causes exponentially more cancers with ultraviolet (UV) radiation each year than medical radiation. In addition to non-melanoma skin cancers, UV radiation likely causes thousands of melanomas each year, many of which are ultimately fatal.

Radon is a decay product of naturally occurring uranium, an element in the earth. This gas is colorless and odorless, so people can't detect it without specific testing equipment. Unfortunately, radon has been shown to cause lung cancer. Most of the studies were done in miners who were working deep below the surface of the earth and were exposed to high levels of radon. While many cases of lung cancer developed in miners who smoked, non-smokers also developed lung cancer as a result of their radon exposure. In fact, it's estimated that among the roughly 10% of lung cancers that occur in nonsmokers today, about half of these cases are the result of radon exposure.

Thankfully, testing for radon has advanced to the point where it can be performed easily and fairly inexpensively today. Many new home buyers are notified of this type of testing prior to purchase. So, when that next infomercial comes on the radio or television touting the new "all natural" cure for some cancer type or other disease, think about the sun...and radon.

Other Home and Work Exposures

The classic example of a product or chemical in the home or workplace causing cancer is asbestos. People who are exposed to asbestos have an increased risk of lung cancer in general, especially if they smoke. In addition, a fairly uncommon type of lung cancer called mesothelioma is caused directly in most cases by asbestos exposure. While mesothelioma can occur in nonsmokers, people who smoke after asbestos exposure have an exponentially increased risk, including for lung cancer in general. Advertisements from attorneys' offices fill newspapers, radio, and television, pleading with people that if they've been exposed to asbestos, "Please call our offices." These lawyers know that if they have a client with a history of asbestos exposure who develops mesothelioma, their case is virtually guaranteed to be a winner. Thankfully, safety agencies have been fairly successful in monitoring removal of most asbestos in existing older homes and buildings, so that future generations should have minimal exposure.

Unfortunately, the list of known or probable cancer-causing chemicals currently in existence is extensive. It's too long, in fact, to be discussed here in any meaningful way. Interested readers are referred again to the "Report on Carcinogens, Eleventh Edition," published by the U.S. Department of Health and Human Services, for an exhaustive list.

Conclusions

There are plenty of risks and threats in life. Some of these are within our control and some aren't. People who care about reducing their risk of a cancer diagnosis need not spend much time or effort on the process, as long as they make a few key decisions wisely. Telling someone who's already reading a book about cancer prevention to avoid using tobacco products is like preaching to the church choir. However, it bears mentioning that hounding close family members and friends to quit usually pays dividends also. While they might not admit it openly, most smokers do care, and many want to quit. They only need the right incentive and a little help.

The few known cancer-causing viruses can be avoided largely by making good choices in the bedroom (or better yet, beforehand!). Parents of 9- to 26-year-olds as well as young adults already out on their own should strongly consider receiving the HPV vaccine. Abstinence is an excellent first line of defense, but backup protection against a possible life-threatening cancer diagnosis is wise. Medical treatments that have cancer-causing potential (albeit small in absolute terms) come in two main types: essential and nonessential. If a cancer requires chemotherapy and/or RT to increase the chance for cure now, then the current benefits generally greatly outweigh the risks of developing another cancer years later as a result of treatment. Nonessential medical treatments that may increase the risk of certain cancer types should be an opportunity to strengthen the doctor-patient relationship with a thorough discussion of risks and benefits.

Most readers who grew up with caring parents recognize the need to minimize sun exposure on the skin. Deadly melanomas as well as the more common nonmelanoma types of skin cancer are much more likely after excessive sun exposure over years, particularly starting at a young age. Ensure that radon levels in and around the home are safe by testing if necessary. Lastly, at home and at work, try to minimize exposures to potentially harmful chemicals. It seems that new studies regarding cancer risks are published each month. In the meantime, common sense goes a long way.

FUEL UP YOUR DEFENSE

One of the best pieces of advice that I received during my medical training was to develop a comfort level with being able to admit when I didn't know something. After completing four years of college, four years of medical school, three to six years of residency, then often a specialty fellowship for another year or two, many doctors find this advice very difficult to follow. While I'm confident in my knowledge about various aspects of cancer, I'm admittedly no expert in the field of nutrition. In fact, I learned more about nutrition during my extracurricular activities than I did throughout my entire medical training.

Over the past decade, I decided to make a transition from aging soccer player to long-distance runner and triathlete. Before long, my goals in the field of endurance sports became loftier (and longer). When making the leap from shorter-distance races to marathons and long-distance triathlons, the importance of nutrition suddenly became much more meaningful in my life. At the same time, I began to delve deeper into the impact of nutrition on my patients.

In my humble opinion, most medical schools don't provide future doctors enough formal instruction about the impact of nutrition on general health. Specifically, there's little discussion about the role that diet plays in minimizing the risk of chronic diseases, including life-threatening illnesses like cancer. Readers who have primary doctors that are knowledgeable about nutrition and are able to share that knowledge should consider themselves very fortunate.

Most unfortunately, however, there's a vast amount of misinformation splattered throughout lots of Web sites and in print about foods to eat for cancer prevention or risk reduction. What should you believe? Which sources are credible? Perhaps most importantly, where's the data?! Plenty of people make grand claims about the power of various food products, herbal mixtures, and supplements to improve health. Sadly, the majority of these products either haven't been studied or they've been studied but found to have no proven protective effect against cancer. Modern snake oil salesmen still prey on people's fears, hopes, and misconceptions. Some sound very convincing and authoritative with claims of cancer prevention. Buyers beware!

Other lower life forms market their products to patients who already have a cancer diagnosis. These patients may be struggling through side effects of cancer treatments that have been proven effective, including surgery, radiation therapy, chemotherapy, or other newer biologic therapies. During these difficult times, less-educated patients are particularly vulnerable to suggestions of "all natural" miracle cures. As one of my old bosses liked to say, "Show me the data!"

Many effective anti-cancer medications and other medical treatments have been "discovered" thanks to naturally occurring plant or animal products. Undoubtedly, researchers and scientists will continue to find gifts in nature with potent medicinal qualities. However, if and/or when there's a magic pill or single food product that guarantees cancer prevention or cure, rest assured that the scientific and medical professionals will be thrilled! That information will be widely and rapidly available. Until that time, it's critical to have a basic understanding of the often complex relationship between cancer risk and nutrition.

Throughout the remainder of this chapter, the impact of dietary or nutritional modification on the risk of developing the most common cancers will be discussed. While a tremendous amount of research has been done regarding the optimal nutrition for patients who already have cancer, the discussion here is limited to reducing risk of a cancer diagnosis in healthy patients. There's also a tremendous amount of existing information about the impact of dietary factors on growth of cancer cells in the laboratory. However, as is the case with many promising new medications, what may look like a home run in the Petri dish or laboratory rodent is frequently a foul ball in the human body. For this reason, the review in this chapter focuses on major studies that have evaluated cancer risk reduction in real people; thousands and thousands of real people!

Nutrition and Breast Cancer Prevention

Breast cancer is the most commonly diagnosed cancer in women in the United States (other than nonmelanoma skin cancer), at about 200,000 cases per year. Among the most common cancers diagnosed overall, breast cancer receives a large proportion of federal cancer research funding. Perhaps it's for this reason that the effect of dietary changes on the risk of breast cancer has been most extensively studied. Despite these studies, however, many questions remain.

The amount or percentage of calories from dietary fat has long been thought to influence breast cancer risk. While a couple of these studies have suggested a correlation, the weight of evidence favors no clear relationship between dietary fat and the risk of developing breast cancer. The largest of these studies, the Women's Health Initiative (WHI) Randomized Controlled Dietary Modification Trial, included nearly 50,000 postmenopausal female participants. In a randomized controlled trial (RCT), half of the participants are chosen at random to receive a treatment or intervention while the other half usually receive a placebo (no intervention) or a different treatment. In the WHI trial, half of the women were randomized to follow a low-fat diet while the other half received no dietary instruction. Fewer breast cancers developed in the group that was actively dieting than the control group (655 versus 1,072). However, the difference didn't reach statistical significance over the eight-year follow-up of these women. So, while women who eat less dietary fat (and/or total calories) may possibly have a lower risk of breast cancer, the impact is so small that a study of 50,000 women failed to show a statistical difference.

It seems logical that an increase in fruits and vegetables might decrease the risk of cancer, since they provide valuable micronutrients. The predominant theory is that antioxidants such as beta-carotene (a form of vitamin A), vitamin C, and vitamin E prevent cellular damage. They're thought to improve our body's own immune system in this way. However, the reality of the benefit of antioxidants as anticancer agents remains far from definite. In fact, the overwhelming weight of evidence indicates no significant relationship between fruit and vegetable consumption and breast cancer prevention.

There are a couple of smaller studies from Japan and Italy that appear to show a protective benefit from flavonoids, a class of phytochemicals (actually plant pigments) that are found in certain fruits and vegetables. Foods containing types of flavonoids include berries, apples, pears, tomatoes, onions, some beans, green tea, and wine. While flavonoids are present in both red and white wines, the levels are generally higher in red wines.

Most of the remaining medical literature regarding the impact of nutrition changes on breast cancer risk involves a smattering of studies on various dietary factors. Vitamin D, for instance, when taken at greater than 800 IU (international units) daily, was found to be protective against breast cancer among the 34,000-plus postmenopausal participants in the Iowa Women's Health Study. Increased calcium from dairy products also appeared to correlate with a decreased risk of breast cancer in a French study. Soy, on the other hand, didn't appear to significantly decrease risk among a large group of Japanese women.

There are no clear, consistent benefits to other food products for breast cancer prevention in the medical literature. For an exhaustive review, the American Institute for Cancer Research's 2007 report titled "Food, Nutrition, Physical Activity and the Prevention of Cancer: A Global Perspective" is a good resource.

Nutrition and Gastrointestinal (GI) Cancer Prevention

If what people eat and drink affects their risk of developing cancer, it makes sense that the most direct impact would be on cancers within the GI system. While cancer may develop within virtually any organ in the GI system, most of the medical literature has focused on two specific areas: cancers of the upper GI tract and colorectal cancer (CRC). Among cancer specialists, cancers of the mouth, throat, and larynx (voice box) are generally labeled together as "head and neck cancers." However, since the mouth is the anatomic and physiologic beginning of the GI tract, these potential cancer sites are included with the upper GI tract here.

The mouth and throat are initially exposed to the effects of what we consume, both food and drink, and are at risk for cancer. Potent carcinogens (cancer-causing agents) like tobacco smoke and the human papilloma virus (HPV) have been found to be responsible for the vast majority of squamous cell cancers of the head and neck (HNSCC). However, a handful of large studies have investigated the effects of nutrition on the risk of developing HNSCC. Two important reports came from Italy. One was a large prospective case-control study. In these types of studies, the cases (people who have cancer) are compared with the controls (people who don't have cancer), usually with respect to a specific question. The other report was a meta-analysis of multiple trials. Because of the seemingly inconsistent results of individual studies, researchers will often perform a massive "study of studies" called a meta-analysis, which evaluates data on thousands of individual patients from multiple studies together. In both reports, groups who ate more fruits and vegetables had a decreased rate of oral and pharyngeal (throat) cancer. In regard to cancer of the larynx, two other large European case-control studies revealed an increased risk for people who ate a relatively high amount of meat, and a decreased risk for people who ate more fruits and vegetables. Vegetable fiber appeared to be more protective against larynx cancer than fruit fiber in one of these studies. In summary, people who consistently eat more fresh fruits and vegetables appear to be at less risk for cancers of the mouth, throat, and voice box. One should also keep in mind, however, that the relative protective effect of diet is easily negated by the harmful effect of cigarette smoking. Eat all the fruits and veggies that you like, but if you smoke, you're still placing yourself at high risk for multiple types of cancer, including HNSCC.

The other main components of the upper GI tract are the esophagus and stomach. Cancers of the esophagus are usually either SCCs (upper to middle) or adenocarcinomas (lower and/or extending into the junction with the stomach). Squamous cell cancers generally arise from superficial parts of the body such as the skin, genitalia, or mucosal covering of the upper GI tract or anus. On the other hand, adenocarcinomas are glandular cancers that arise from deeper within the body. The vast majority of cancers of the breast, prostate, and colon are adenocarcinomas. As one might expect, the main causes of these two types of cancer in the esophagus and stomach are different.

The upper esophagus can be thought of as an extension of the pharynx or throat. These organs have the same type of lining and are exposed to similar insults on a regular basis. Tobacco smoke, alcohol, and other chronic irritants are the source of most of these cancers, with the major exception being throat cancers that can also be due to human papillomavirus (HPV) infection. It should come as no surprise then, that irritating foods and drinks have shown a similar relationship, though not as strong. Parts of the world with the highest number of cases of SCC of the esophagus include parts of the Middle and Far East, where people regularly consume hot, spicy foods and beverages as part of the culture. Clear correlations have been shown between consumption of spicy foods, including salted meats as well as hot drinks and an increased risk of developing esophageal SCC in Taiwan, Uruguay, and several other countries. A decreased risk has been shown for people who eat more fruit, vegetables, and fish.

Adenocarcinomas of the stomach, particularly at the gastroesophageal junction, have been diagnosed much more frequently in the United States over the past 10-20 years. They're often the result of chronic reflux of stomach contents into the lower esophagus that may result in a condition called Barrett's esophagus. Multiple studies have evaluated the role of specific foods and micronutrients in the development of these cancers. The European Prospective Investigation into Cancer and Nutrition (EPIC) cohort study was a massive undertaking involving hundreds of thousands of people in ten countries that gathered huge amounts of data about nutrition's impact on cancer and other diseases. An increased risk of stomach cancer was shown to correlate with increased intake of processed and red meat, decreased intake of fruits and vegetables, and decreased adherence to a Mediterranean diet. Multiple other studies appear to confirm the protective effect of high fruit and vegetable intake, as well as the increased risk for those who eat large amounts of processed meats. According to two studies from China, micronutrients associated with a possible decreased risk of esophageal and stomach cancers include retinol, beta carotene, vitamin E, and selenium. Lastly, two negative studies for adenocarcinomas of the esophagus and stomach were reported regarding the influence of carbonated soft drinks and soy products. The authors thought that carbonated drinks might increase risk and soy products might decrease it, but their hypotheses were unproven in both cases.

The most common GI cancer is colorectal (CRC). Diagnosed in about 150,000 patients in the United States annually, CRC will eventually be the cause of death for about a third of these patients. Because CRC is so common and because most of what we eat and drink directly contacts the bowel in some way, the impact of dietary changes on CRC has been widely studied. Major studies in the United States, Europe, and other countries have demonstrated common themes, though not universally similar results. The EPIC study from Europe involving approximately 500,000 people revealed a direct correlation between intake of red meat and CRC, as well as a protective effect for the regular consumption of fish. The National Cancer Institute-AARP Diet and Health Study, also with roughly 500,000 participants, revealed a similar correlation between red meat consumption and an increased risk of CRC.

Studies of the effect of fruits and vegetable consumption on CRC risk have been more conflicting. The WHI Dietary Modification Trial involving almost fifty thousand women chose half of the women at random to receive dietary changes aimed at decreasing dietary fat and increasing servings of fruits, vegetables, and grains. While there was a trend toward more CRC cases among women who didn't change their diet (279 cases versus 201 cases), there was no clear statistical benefit to the group of women who consumed a diet containing more fruits and vegetables. These results are very similar to those for the effect of fruit and vegetable consumption on breast cancer prevention. There may be a benefit for people who routinely eat more fruits and vegetables, but the benefit is likely small since this study of fifty thousand women failed to show a statistical difference. Nevertheless, since it's clear that red, processed meats increased risk for CRC and there are many health benefits to eating fresh fruits and vegetables, a regular diet adhering to these two principles seems wise.

Nutrition and Gynecologic (GYN) Cancer Prevention

While not the most common GYN cancer, ovarian cancer is the most deadly in the United States. Not surprisingly, it's also been the most studied in terms of its association with nutritional factors. One of the largest trials was the WHI Dietary Modification Randomized Controlled Trial. Half of the women in the study were asked to limit fat to 20% or less of their caloric intake and to increase their intake of fruits and vegetables. A slight decrease in ovarian cancer was noted, although no benefit for uterine cancer prevention was seen. Smaller studies in Canada and Italy revealed a direct correlation between cholesterol and red meat intake and the risk of ovarian cancer. A diet rich in fish and vegetables decreased ovarian cancer risk in the latter study. However, the massive EPIC study, which included over 300,000 female participants across the continent, failed to show a significant protective effect of high fruit and vegetable intake. The Nurses' Health Study, another massive undertaking that included over 60,000 women, did reveal a protective effect for ovarian cancer among women who consumed relatively high amounts of certain types of flavonoids, antioxidants found in diverse food groups. An Italian study found similar protective effects for flavonols and isoflavones. A mild effect was found for beta-carotene in a meta-analysis performed by researchers at the Marshfield Clinic in Wisconsin. Thus, women who want to minimize their risk of ovarian cancer may do so (at least slightly) by minimizing red meat consumption and regularly eating fresh fruits and vegetables, including those containing flavonoids.

While studied less extensively than ovarian cancer, uterine cancer risk has been found to correlate with increased fat, animal protein, cholesterol, and total energy (calorie) intake. A meta-analysis on the effect of vitamin D and calcium on endometrial cancer risk failed to show a significant association. Thus, the diet recommended to minimize ovarian cancer risk may also serve to decrease uterine cancer risk.

Nutrition and Lung Cancer Prevention

Lung cancer is exceedingly common and the leading cancer killer in the United States and the world. While the vast majority of cases are caused by the direct carcinogenic effects of smoking tobacco, a small proportion of lung cancer occurs in nonsmokers. Moreover, some smokers appear to be more prone to developing lung cancer than others. Several major studies have evaluated the role of dietary changes on lung cancer prevention. The EPIC study, for instance, revealed a significant protective effect for fruit consumption, although eating more vegetables didn't appear to help. A French study restricted to nonsmokers found a clear protective effect for vegetables, including tomatoes, carrots, and lettuce. They also found that fruit consumption was protective for squamous cell and small cell types of lung cancer. While the Beta-Carotene and Retinol Efficacy (CARET) trial revealed a potential unexpected increase in lung cancer risk with beta-carotene intake, researchers found a protective effect for certain fruits and cruciferous vegetables, such as broccoli and cauliflower. Several studies on the effects of beta-carotene, antioxidants in general, selenium, and multivitamin and mineral supplementation have all failed to show a significant protective effect against lung cancer. Lastly, in the EPIC study, there was no clear effect of alcohol consumption on lung cancer risk. The bottom line to avoid lung cancer remains avoiding tobacco products. However, people who eat more fresh fruits and vegetables regularly may have a lower risk than those who don't.

Nutrition and Prostate Cancer Prevention

Unfortunately, cancer may develop within virtually any organ in the genitourinary (GU) tract. However, the vast majority of literature regarding risk reduction for these cancers through dietary changes focuses on cancer of the prostate. It's the most common cancer of the GU system, diagnosed in over 200,000 men annually in the United States. Many dietary studies have been completed that evaluate the role of different food groups on prostate cancer prevention. Unfortunately, the results of many of these major studies appear contradictory.

The effect of dairy products has been extensively evaluated. Dairy protein and calcium from dairy products were shown to correlate with an increased risk of prostate cancer in both the massive EPIC study, as well as smaller studies from France and Greece. However, in two other major reports, the Alpha Tocopherol Beta-Carotene Cancer Prevention (ATBC) Study and the Prostate, Lung, Colorectal, and Ovarian Cancer Screening Trials, the association of dairy and calcium intake with development of prostate cancer was weak at best.

There may be a benefit for men with higher intakes of vegetables, especially those rich in Vitamin C, although these studies were fairly small. In fact, it appears that there are many more negative studies about the role of dietary changes on the development of prostate cancer than there are positive ones. Among the dietary elements that haven't been proven to correlate with prostate cancer risk are: total meat intake (though "very well done" meat may be risky due to mutagenic heterocyclic amines), lycopene (found in tomatoes), alcohol, fiber, vitamin E, and multivitamins. In fact, the National Institutes of Health – AARP Diet and Health Study found that men with "excessive multivitamin use" actually had an increased risk of developing advanced or fatal prostate cancer. Lastly, the role of selenium supplementation to decrease prostate cancer risk remains in doubt, with studies showing a potential protective benefit, but likely limited to men who had baseline low selenium levels in their blood.

For those who wish to delve extensively into details of specific reports regarding the potential relationship between nutrition and prostate cancer prevention, I recommend the 2007 expert report from the American Institute of Cancer Research titled "Food, Nutrition, Physical Activity and the Prevention of Cancer: a Global Perspective." In summary though, no specific dietary modification has been shown to significantly decrease the risk of prostate cancer.

TAKE THE BALL BY THE HORNS

No, the title of this chapter doesn't contain a typo. My wife is the queen of the mixed metaphor. On more than a few occasions, she's had our friends in stitches with her uncanny ability to mix words and phrases. However, "Take the Ball by the Horns" wasn't a Jill Maguire original. It's my way of conveying that people who truly care about reducing their risk of cancer need to take an active, maybe even aggressive role in the process. For many, it may not mean literally taking a ball out to play a regular game of soccer or basketball. Regular walking, running, biking, swimming, or other vigorous physical activity will serve the purpose. Many people are able to get that type of activity while they work. Most of us, however, need to carve out leisure time for the purpose. As with many aspects of life, if it's important enough, we'll find the time!

Can a book about health improvement truly be complete without a chapter on exercise? Most folks love it or hate it. They find it a source of pleasure and stress relief or dread it like a form of torture. Some guys look forward to their weekend ballgame, and may even prepare for it by running and lifting weights two or three days during the week. Others look forward to sitting on the couch to watch a ballgame. Some women look forward to their morning run as the highlight of their day, a time when they feel most awake and alive. Others look forward to sleeping that extra hour, too exhausted to even think about regular exercise. Regardless of one's emotions about exercise, however, most people acknowledge "it's good for you." In fact, for many who don't get pleasure from their exercise, the only reason that they get up early or head to the gym after a long day at the office is because they feel they're sustaining or improving their health. Most people think about the obvious benefit to their heart from regular cardiovascular activity. Some are concerned about maintaining or improving their appearance, slimming a waistline, or increasing muscle mass. Few, however, think about cancer prevention as a reason to exercise.

Cancer development is often a complex process. Multiple factors act together within our bodies to cause cancer, so it seems wise to have multiple methods to combat them. Avoiding known carcinogens and being vigilant about nutrition are critical, though they may not be sufficient to minimize risk. Regular physical activity can be viewed as an added level of insurance against a cancer diagnosis.

This chapter reviews the best scientific studies available regarding the role of exercise in reducing cancer risk. The focus is on the "big four": breast cancer, colorectal cancer, lung cancer, and prostate cancer. Some of the results may be surprising.

Exercise and Breast Cancer Prevention

The impact of physical activity on reducing cancer risk has been more extensively studied for breast cancer than for most other types. As was the case with nutritional studies, the best studies of exercise and breast cancer risk are cohort or case control studies. Cohort studies look forward in time (prospectively) over a long time, following a large group or groups of people. Case-control studies compare two groups of people: one that has the specific problem or disease in question (in this case, breast cancer) and one that doesn't. In the specific case of exercise and its relationship to breast cancer prevention, the medical literature can be further split into two main topics: physical activity itself and its impact on female hormones.

Several major studies have evaluated the role of physical activity and breast cancer prevention. The first was the Nurses' Health Study, which enrolled thousands of women 30 to 55 years old in Massachusetts beginning in the late 1970s. These women were followed over decades and given questionnaires about various aspects of their life, including their amount and type of physical activity. Among those enrolled and followed over 16 years, more than 3,000 women developed breast cancer. The investigators found that women who reported moderate to vigorous physical activity for seven or more hours per week had a significantly decreased risk of breast cancer (about 20% less) than women who reported less than one hour of the same type of activity. A couple of smaller European studies confirmed more of a benefit to moderate or vigorous activity over light activity. In one of these studies, the protective effect for exercise appeared to be independent of family history, menopausal status, or body mass index.

Many researchers have investigated whether there's a dose-response to the protective effect of exercise against the risk of breast or other cancer types. In other words, is a lot of exercise better than a little? When they performed a massive analysis of 34 case-control studies and 28 cohort studies that had been published in the medical literature, two Canadian researchers found that 47 of the 62 studies (76%) showed a decrease in breast cancer risk associated with increased physical activity. Among the 33 studies that evaluated for dose-response (whether more exercise was better), 28 studies (85%) came to the conclusion that it was.

The benefits of exercise in decreasing breast cancer risk appear to apply to both black and white women. The Women's Contraceptive and Reproductive Experience Study was a case-control study that included over 9,000 women, roughly half of whom had a diagnosis of breast cancer. About a third of patients were black and two-thirds were white. This study showed that both black and white women who were more physically active had a decreased risk of breast cancer compared to women who were relatively inactive.

Because it's widely known that female hormones play a key role in the development of breast cancer for many women, other researchers have investigated how physical activity affects sex hormone levels. Prior studies had shown that increased estradiol levels and decreased sex-hormone binding globulin levels, for instance, were associated with an increased risk of breast cancer. Two recent trials which randomized sedentary (relatively inactive) women to vigorous exercise for a few hours per week versus no increased activity or only stretching found that the exercise significantly affected the levels of these important sex hormones. The investigators concluded that the protective effect of exercise against breast cancer risk is likely due, at least in part, to its effects on sex hormone levels.

Exercise and Colorectal Cancer Prevention

The relationship between exercise and colorectal cancer (CRC) prevention appears clear. Some people, due to unfortunate genetics, will be at high risk for CRC and their options for risk reduction are few. However, risk factors for developing CRC in most of the population are "modifiable." They can be changed or altered if the individual is motivated to do so. Virtually everyone is aware of the impact of diet on the risk of CRC. Some people also know that alcohol and tobacco use can increase the risk of CRC. However, few people realize that physical activity level is also important. Many studies have come to the same conclusion independently. Perhaps the largest was a meta-analysis performed by Australian investigators that included 103 different cohort studies. This massive study showed a clear negative impact of alcohol, tobacco, red meat, diabetes, and obesity. The researchers also confirmed a positive, protective effect of physical activity against the risk of CRC.

A few other major studies showed that both occupational and recreational activity levels may be important for CRC risk. Researchers from Norway followed over 60,000 men and women who had undergone screening in the 1970s and found that those with highest occupational and recreational activity levels had the lowest rates of developing CRC. A group from the National Cancer Institute (NCI) showed that light occupational activity was helpful, moderate to heavy activity at work was better, but leisure activity didn't correlate with CRC risk. Lastly, the Nurses' Health Study confirmed the benefit of increased physical activity and leaner body mass index for women to protect against CRC.

Exercise and Lung Cancer Prevention

Readers who smoke should make quitting priority No. 1 (as well as priority No. 2 through No. 10) for lung cancer prevention. However, those who can't or won't quit smoking cigarettes or using other tobacco products do have some other options to minimize the relative risk of developing lung cancer. One of these, believe it or not, is exercise. Investigators from Harvard University evaluated almost 14,000 male alumni between the 1970s and 1990s. Among this huge group of men, 245 developed lung cancer. By looking at multiple potential factors, the researchers found that activities such as walking, climbing stairs, or participating in other physical activity of "moderate intensity" significantly decreased the risk of lung cancer for both smokers and nonsmokers.

The Alpha-Tocopherol, Beta-Carotene Cancer Prevention (ATBC) Study was one of the few studies that failed to show a protective effect for exercise against the risk of lung cancer. However, among the 27,000 smokers included, those who were younger did appear to have a small benefit which was probably negated (statistically) by the lack of effect of exercise on older smokers.

There appears to be a dose-response for the amount of exercise protecting against lung cancer also. A meta-analysis of reports published between 1966 and 2003 by investigators at the National Cancer Institute revealed that an increase in leisure-time activity correlated with a decrease in lung cancer risk. High levels of vigorous activity were more protective than moderate activity levels.

Exercise and Prostate Cancer Prevention

Can exercise make a man's prostate healthier? The answer is...maybe, but studies are conflicting. A couple of major trials have shown a benefit. The ATBC Cancer Prevention Study included over 29,000 men, of whom 317 developed prostate cancer. Investigators evaluated activity type and intensity and found a protective effect against prostate cancer from being physically active. Men who walked regularly had a clear benefit over those who were sedentary. So, at least in this massive study, exercise didn't have to be too strenuous; just walking helped.

The European Prospective Investigation into Cancer and Nutrition (EPIC) cohort study included about 128,000 men ages 20 to 97 years. Almost 2,500 of these men developed prostate cancer. When different types of exercise were evaluated, regular participation in walking, gardening, cycling, and sports activity failed to show a protective effect against prostate cancer. However, men who reported a high level of physical exertion at their jobs had a significantly decreased risk of advanced prostate cancer.

A couple of case-control studies have also shown a benefit to physical activity in decreasing prostate cancer risk. One study in China revealed that men who participated in moderate physical activity had less risk of prostate cancer. They also found a dose-response such that less activity was less protective. A larger Italian study that included 1,300 cases and almost 1,500 control patients revealed that men from age 30 to age 59 who engaged in more strenuous activity at work had a significantly decreased risk of prostate cancer.

Unfortunately though, the results of all studies on this topic aren't consistently positive. Two other massive studies failed to show a clear benefit to physical activity in decreasing prostate cancer risk. The Health Professionals Follow-up Study included almost 48,000 men ranging in age from 40 to 75 years. The researchers evaluated the role of total physical activity, both vigorous and nonvigorous. They found no clear relationship with the development of prostate cancer, though there was a suggestion that metastatic prostate cancer (cancer that's spread to distant sites and is generally incurable) was less likely to occur in men who performed vigorous exercise regularly.

The Physicians' Health Study was a prospective (forward-looking) randomized controlled trial (RCT) that enrolled over 22,000 men and evaluated the impact of aspirin and beta-carotene on the risks of heart attack, stroke, and cancer. Over a follow-up period of 11 years, almost 1,000 of these men developed prostate cancer. The researchers found no association between exercise "vigorous enough to work up a sweat" and the risk of developing prostate cancer.

Because the results of individual studies have been conflicting, several groups of researchers have performed meta-analyses to evaluate the relationship between exercise and prostate cancer prevention. One report looked at 14 studies, the second looked at 24 studies, and the last evaluated 27 total studies. While the majority showed a protective effect of physical activity against a diagnosis of prostate cancer, many did not. The bottom line currently appears to be that while a benefit may exist, it's likely fairly small.

Conclusions

Exercise appears to decrease the risk of the most common deadly cancers in general. Physical activity decreases breast cancer risk, at least partly by affecting levels of sex hormones in the body. There's clearly a protective effect of exercise against developing CRC. The risk of lung cancer may be decreased somewhat by regular exercise in younger smokers. Studies on the relationship between physical activity and the risk of prostate cancer are conflicting. If exercise has any protective effect against the development of prostate cancer, it's likely quite weak.

THE NEXT BEST THING

Many people will say, "Doc, I don't smoke. I eat a healthy diet. I exercise regularly. How did I get cancer?" Active lifestyle decisions and choices like these can be difficult to make. They involve thought, preparation, and, for most people, some sacrifice. They're critical to minimizing the risk of a cancer diagnosis. Unfortunately, they're not sufficient for cancer prevention altogether. In fact, complete prevention of all cancers isn't possible, at least not as of this writing in 2010. Cancer "risk reduction" is probably a more appropriate term than cancer prevention.

The first few, most difficult steps in the risk reduction process are the active choices that one makes to minimize harmful exposures, optimize nutrition, and maintain a reasonable physical activity level. These decisions maintain the body's first line of defense, the immune system. Despite best intentions and efforts, however, many men and women will still find themselves facing a cancer diagnosis. In this situation, it's much better to be faced with a potentially curable cancer than one that's already metastasized (spread; generally incurable). The currently available cancer screening tests that have been proven to detect several common types early are a second line of defense against dying of an incurable cancer. In most cases, if a cancer is diagnosed at an early stage, then the chances for cure remain high. The next best thing to cancer prevention is early detection!

There are several critical requirements that a medical screening test must meet in order to be effective and worthwhile. First, the test needs to address a significant public health problem for which there's a cure if/when the disease is detected early. Second, it must be able to detect the disease not only early but also across the majority of the population that's being screened. When that criterion is met, the test is also more likely to be cost effective. While cost of a test isn't the number one priority, it's still important. Last but not least, the screening test should be safe to administer and widely available. It doesn't do society much good if only the wealthy or privileged are able to undergo the test (or the treatment, for that matter!).

There are multiple medical articles and trials testing the role of various cancer screening tests. Generally, the most important and influential of these trials are called randomized controlled trials (RCTs). In the case of screening studies, these RCTs usually involve tens or hundreds of thousands of people. Half of those enrolled receive the screening test and half don't. The people are then followed by their doctors and researchers over many years. A portion of people in both groups (screened and unscreened) will develop the type of cancer in question, and some of these patients in both groups will die of their disease. The researchers then compare the death rates in the control group versus the screened group in order to determine if the screening test was successful.

Some general doctors review these individual studies periodically in order to help them have more informed discussions with their patients. However, the cancer screening recommendations that most U.S. physicians follow are from "The American Cancer Society (ACS) Guidelines for the Early Detection of Cancer," which were updated in 2010. Readers are encouraged to review this short document in its entirety. To do so, go online to www.cancer. org. The guidelines include recommendations for breast cancer, cervical cancer, colorectal cancer, prostate cancer, and endometrial (uterine) cancer. The main recommendation for uterine cancer is to consider endometrial biopsy for high-risk patients. Uterine cancer screening won't be discussed further.

Among the "big four" (the most commonly diagnosed cancers in the United States: breast, lung, colon, and prostate), only lung cancer doesn't have a standard screening test that's been proven effective. Major studies have evaluated chest x-rays and CT scans as cancer screening tests for lung cancer in high-risk populations. However, these scans haven't proven to be effective enough cancer screening tests for widespread use. Patients and their families often question, "Why don't we just do scans on everybody so that we can find cancers early? Is it the insurance companies wanting to save their money?" While there's usually no great love lost between doctors and insurance companies these days, most physicians will point out that widespread screening with certain tests may cause more harm than good for the public. Lung cancer screening with chest CT scans fell into that category, at least until recently. Initial findings from the National Lung Screening Trial (NLST) were just released (www.cancer.gov/nlst/updates). This trial included over 53,000 people ages 55-74 with extensive smoking histories. It tested CXR versus low-dose helical chest CT scans to screen for lung cancer. Patients who received CT screening had a 20% decrease in deaths due to lung cancer compared with those who received CXR screening. Although widespread chest CT screening for lung cancer is not currently ready for primetime, it may well be beneficial for very high-risk patients like those who participated in the trial. Cancer specialists are now anxiously awaiting the final NLST report to study the details.

Some of the ACS recommendations for cancer screening are straightforward, while others leave room for individual choices. In this chapter, the focus is on four potentially life-saving tests: mammography, the prostate specific antigen (PSA) test, the Pap test, and colonoscopy.

Breast Cancer Screening with Mammography

Mammography is diagnostic medical imaging of the breast tissue using radiation and specialized x-ray film. Generally, mammogram images of the breasts are taken from two different views: craniocaudal (CC; from top to bottom) and mediolateral oblique (MLO; at an angle from the middle to the outside of the breast). Further imaging, including close-up views of any suspicious areas, may be requested by the radiologist at the time of the procedure. This doctor then interprets the images and sends a copy of the report to the patient's primary doctor. If the results are suspicious for cancer, then recommendation may be made for repeat imaging (often three to six months) or for immediate surgical consultation for biopsy. If the exam is unremarkable, then the common recommendation is for continued screening once per year.

In the United States, both the ACS and the U.S. Preventive Services Task Force (USPSTF) has provided guidelines for mammography in the role of early detection of breast cancer for many years. These guidelines are based on interpretations of major RCTs whose basic question has been whether mammography decreases deaths due to breast cancer, and, if so, in which groups of women. Some aspects of the guidelines haven't changed, while some have caused controversy dating back 20 years.

There's consensus among the experts on a few aspects of breast cancer screening. Both ultrasound and magnetic resonance imaging (MRI) of the breast are unproven as widespread screening tests. They're helpful for some patients after mammography to evaluate suspicious areas in the breast, but they're not effective screening tests on their own. Neither breast self exam by patients nor clinical breast examination by doctors has been proven effective in the studies that have evaluated them. Since many women have heard for years to do breast exams each month and to see their doctors for an exam each year, this information may be puzzling. The bottom line is that most lumps felt by both patients and doctors won't be malignant (cancerous). Therefore, the majority of these masses that are felt will generate further evaluation, anxiety, costs, and often invasive biopsies that won't lead to an early cancer diagnosis and improved cure rate. However, some will be cancer. Lack of statistical benefit in a medical study does *not* mean that women should disregard any visible or palpable changes that they notice in their breasts. It's very helpful to be attuned to clues such as a new lump, redness, dimpling of the skin, etc., and notify one's doctor. In the author's experience, countless patients have found their cancers early by being in tune, literally in touch, with their bodies.

The only screening tool for breast cancer that's consistently been shown to decrease the risk of death due to breast cancer is mammography. The sensitivity (likelihood of the test being abnormal when cancer is actually there) of mammography is roughly 80%, and the specificity (likelihood of the test being normal when there's actually no cancer there) is 90%. So, although not 100% accurate, mammography is a fairly good screening test. Throughout most areas in the United States where women have reasonable access to health care, the majority are diagnosed with invasive cancer and/or ductal carcinoma in situ (DCIS; preinvasive cancer) solely by mammogram. Most of these patients are asymptomatic (have no symptoms). Neither they nor their doctors felt a lump. Mammography clearly detects many breast cancers earlier than would be possible by physical examination or symptoms alone.

Interpreting mammogram images can be challenging in certain subsets of women. These include women who are younger than 50 years old, have dense breasts, or have had prior surgery, radiation therapy (RT), and/or hormone therapy replacement. Mammography is also much less reliable for detecting lobular carcinoma, though this breast cancer subtype is much less common than ductal carcinoma. However, the majority of women for whom mammography is recommended will have reliable imaging and interpretation.

The ultimate goal of any cancer screening test, including mammography, is whether the test decreases patients' risk of dying of that particular type of cancer. Multiple RCTs have been conducted to answer this important question about mammography. They've been conducted in multiple countries, including Canada, Scotland, Sweden, the United States, and the United Kingdom. Two examples of the strongest of these RCTs are the National Breast Screening Studies (NBSS) 1 and 2 from Canada. Both of these major trials were well designed. However, since they were conducted mainly through the 1980s, one could argue that the results may differ today in light of improvements in mammographic imaging as well as advances in breast cancer treatment. Women in both of these Canadian studies who were diagnosed with breast cancer received appropriate systemic treatments available at that time, including chemotherapy and/or hormones. This fact is important, since death as a result of breast cancer was the main endpoint being evaluated by both studies. All women underwent clinical breast exam, and half were randomized to receive mammography in addition. The NBSS-1 study enrolled women ages 40 to 49, and the NBSS-2 study enrolled women ages 50 to 59. Both of these RCTs showed no significant decrease in breast cancer deaths among women who had regular mammograms. Although the trials from other countries had problems with their design and other shortcomings, almost all of them showed no statistically significant impact of mammography on the risk of death due to breast cancer.

One possible reason that these trials of mammography didn't show a significant decrease in deaths due to breast cancer is that cancers detected by mammograms alone may be more favorable (less aggressive or deadly). At least two studies have revealed that even after accounting for other important factors, such as tumor stage and patient age, breast cancers that are detected by mammogram are more favorable and less life-threatening than those found by the patient or doctor otherwise. These results indicate that tumors found by mammogram alone may have a less aggressive biology than other breast tumors that are able to be seen or felt.

Despite the lack of statistical evidence among historical RCTs for the benefit of mammography, there's been an approximately 25% decrease in the annual number of deaths due to breast cancer between 1990 and 2000 in the United States. During this same time period, the number of women in the United States undergoing mammography increased significantly. However, major advances were also achieved in the systemic treatment of breast cancer. Therefore, an expert panel decided to evaluate the impact of increased screening versus the impact of improvements in treatment on the decrease in the breast cancer death rate. After extensive evaluation and statistical modeling, they concluded that breast cancer screening with mammograms accounted for 28% to 65% of the decrease in deaths due to breast cancer, while treatment improvements accounted for the remainder. So, at least in the opinions of these experts, mammography has been playing a major role in decreasing breast cancer deaths in the United States.

Yet another massive study was recently published that evaluated the effect of screening mammography on breast cancer deaths in Norway. The study included 40,000 women between the ages of 50 and 69 in four groups: one group that received screening and one group that didn't between 1996 and 2005, as well as two groups who were living in screened and unscreened counties between 1986 and 1995 who served as historical controls. While the study revealed a decrease in breast cancer deaths over time, only about 30% of the benefit was due to screening. These results are on the low end of the statistical modeling study in the U.S. (between 28% and 65%) mentioned above. The remainder of the decrease in breast cancer deaths was thought to be due to advances in breast cancer treatment.

Another area of controversy is the appropriate age to begin screening mammography. Several trials have grouped the results of RCTs through meta-analysis. Some have shown a decrease in the rate of deaths from breast cancer when women are screened in their 40s, while others have found that the benefit is limited to women who are screened in their 50s and 60s. These different findings have led to differing current guidelines for women. Some groups recommend that mammography start at age 50, while the ACS continues to recommend doctors initiate discussions with their female patients at age 40. There's no doubt that starting mammography at age 40 will detect more cancers, but the process will result in many more women undergoing biopsies which will be negative. Many of these younger women will have dense breasts, and their mammograms will be challenging to interpret. Since failure to diagnose breast cancer is a leading reason why physicians are sued, more testing will be done rather than less, even when the risk of cancer is small. However, it appears that most women in the United States are comfortable with aggressive screening to detect an occasional cancer among the few, and they are willing to accept the potential harms of invasive negative biopsies in the many.

In summary, mammography has proven to be an effective screening test that allows for early detection of most breast cancers in women who undergo regular testing. It's partially responsible for decreasing deaths due to breast cancer in the United States over the past couple decades. I continue to recommend to most of my female patients that they follow the ACS Guidelines for breast cancer screening. Specifically, I recommend that they consider beginning annual mammograms at age 40, be aware of any noticeable changes in their breasts, and see their primary doctors at least once per year.

Prostate Cancer Screening with the PSA Test

The prostate specific antigen (PSA) test is a simple blood test that detects a specific protein on cells from the prostate gland in a man's body. This total PSA level should be very low in most young, healthy men. However, it often rises a bit with age and may also be elevated with several conditions other than prostate cancer, including infection, inflammation, and benign prostatic hypertrophy (BPH, noncancerous enlargement of the gland). Nevertheless, an elevated PSA test should raise the suspicion of the possibility of prostate cancer and requires further consideration.

If an otherwise healthy man has a PSA above the standard top normal level of 4 nanograms per milliliter (ng/ml) of blood or an abnormal digital rectal exam (DRE), then generally his primary doctor will refer him for consultation with a urologist, a surgical specialist in the treatment of genitourinary tract diseases. The urologist may then perform a transrectal ultrasound with biopsies of the prostate to determine the presence or absence of cancer.

The American Cancer Society (ACS) currently recommends that doctors have conversations about PSA testing with their male patients who have a life expectancy of more than 10 years. These are the men who are most likely to benefit from treatment if they're found to have prostate cancer after biopsy. Men who are at average risk should begin receiving this information at age 50. For those with a PSA greater than 4 ng/ml, biopsy should be discussed. Among a group of "typical" 70 year-old men undergoing PSA testing, roughly one in four (25%) with a PSA greater than 4 ng/ml will be found to have prostate cancer at the time of biopsy. For those with a PSA less than 2.5 ng/ml, the ACS currently recommends less frequent monitoring, with PSA testing once every two years. While some men may have cancer cells in their prostate even with very low PSA blood levels (less than 1 ng/ml), the likelihood is low (about 1%). For those with borderline PSA levels between 2.5 and 4.0 ng/ml, "individualized risk assessment and decision making" is suggested, especially for men at higher risk (see below).

In addition to the total PSA blood level, there are several other factors that may predict for a higher risk of prostate cancer prior to biopsy. Patient factors include age and race. As men get older, the risk of prostate cancer rises. Black men have a higher risk of developing more aggressive disease at younger ages than white men. Men with a family history of prostate cancer also have a higher baseline risk of disease. The ACS, as well as the American Urological Association (AUA), recommends that doctors initiate discussion of risks and benefits of PSA testing in these high-risk patients beginning at age 40 to 45. The decision between initiation at age 40 versus 45 years old depends on the degree of increased risk.

There are a few laboratory parameters in addition to the baseline total PSA level that may provide further information. The rate of rise of the PSA level over time compared to prior values, often referred to as the "PSA velocity," is another reasonable indicator of tumor biology. One might anticipate that a man whose PSA climbed from 1.5 to 3.0 ng/ml over the course of a year would be much more likely to have prostate cancer than a man whose PSA rose from 2.9 to 3.0 ng/ml over the same time. However, research has indicated that the PSA velocity isn't independently helpful in predicting the presence of cancer over and above the absolute PSA value. Other parameters that urologists use in some cases include the level of free PSA (versus total PSA) and the PSA density. Although these tests may be useful for deciding about prostate biopsy in individual patients with borderline PSA values, their benefit in large studies is minimal beyond that of the basic PSA test. Lastly, a recent report that used a panel of four markers, including total PSA, free PSA, intact PSA, and another protein, appears to show some promise for potentially reducing the number of invasive prostate biopsies performed, while missing very few aggressive cancers.

Like mammograms and other cancer screening tests, there are potential harms associated with PSA testing. Perhaps the greatest of these is called "overdiagnosis." Basically, a large proportion of men will have very early, low-risk prostate cancers diagnosed by PSA testing that wouldn't have otherwise been discovered or hurt them during their lives. Estimates for overdiagnosis range between about 20% and 40% of men who receive PSA testing. Many of these men will opt for aggressive treatment with surgery, brachytherapy (a type of internal radiation treatment), or external beam, intensity modulated radiation therapy. Patients with low-risk disease will have a 90% cure rate with these therapies, but a small portion will be significantly harmed by side effects. They wouldn't otherwise have been harmed if their cancer hadn't been discovered solely via PSA testing. Another risk of PSA screening is failure to diagnose the cancer, since the test isn't 100% accurate. Lastly, some studies have shown a significant long-term increase in anxiety after an elevated PSA test, even after biopsies reveal no cancer. Clearly, PSA testing isn't totally harmless. However, when limited to the correct population of informed men, its potential benefits outweigh its risks in my opinion.

The PSA test has had an effect on prostate cancer diagnosis that's similar to the effect of mammography on breast cancer diagnosis over the past 20 years. In the past, when mammograms were performed less often, breast cancers were detected in later stages more frequently. Over the time period of progressive widespread use of mammography, the number of deaths due to breast cancer decreased in the United States. Similarly, as the PSA blood test became more widespread from 1990 to 2000 to 2010, more prostate cancers were detected in earlier stages. A higher proportion of men had low-risk disease, and an improved chance for cure. Experts at one academic institution saw an increase in the proportion of low-risk disease from 28% to 46% between the early 1990s and mid-2000s. While PSA screening has become more common, deaths from prostate cancer have become less common, declining about 4% per year in the United States during this time period. Was this decline a direct result of enhanced PSA screening, improvements in treatment, or both?!

Ultimately, the critical question to be answered about the value of PSA testing is whether it prevents deaths. Has the rise of PSA testing over the past 20 years contributed to a decline in deaths due to prostate cancer, and, if so, how much? Two major RCTs designed to address this question were recently published, but their methods and results were quite different. The Prostate, Lung, Colorectal, and Ovarian (PLCO) Cancer Screening Trial in the United States enrolled 77,000 men ages 55 to 74, half of whom were randomized to receive yearly screening with both DRE and PSA testing. Unfortunately, a very large proportion of men in the PLCO study who were randomized to receive no screening did actually have PSA testing performed, thereby clouding the results. This study revealed no decrease in the death rate due to prostate cancer in the men who were randomized to screening after an average follow-up of seven years. Quite to the contrary, the European Randomized Study of Screening for Prostate Cancer (ERSPC) revealed a 20% decrease in the rate of deaths due to prostate cancer over an average follow-up of nine years. This trial enrolled 162,000 men ages 55 to 69 who were screened mainly with PSA only once every four years (not annually with DRE as in the U.S. study). Patients in the ERSPC study had biopsies recommended if their PSA was 3 ng/ml or higher, rather than at a threshold of 4 ng/ml as used in the PLCO study. Also, more than 85% of men in the ERSPC study who had an abnormal PSA underwent recommended biopsies, as opposed to less than 50% of men in the PLCO trial. These discrepancies within the trials may at least partially account for the differing results.

In summary, the PSA is a simple and effective blood test that leads to early detection of prostate cancer and may improve a man's chance for cure. It's probably been a significant contributor to the decrease in prostate cancer deaths in this country over the past 15 years. Beginning at age 40 to 50 (depending upon individual risk), healthy men should discuss the risks and benefits of regular PSA testing with their doctors. Once testing is started, PSA levels should be rechecked every year to two years, assuming no other health changes. Among men who are very elderly or whose lives are limited due to other severe illnesses, very few will benefit from PSA testing.

Cervical Cancer Screening with the Pap Test

As opposed to mammography and PSA testing, both of which have controversial aspects, the Pap test is nearly universally accepted as an excellent screening test for cervical cancer. Dr. George Papanicolaou was a pathologist working at Cornell University in New York. He was viewing cells under a microscope that were taken from a smear or swab of fluid from a patient's vagina, when he discovered the presence of cancer cells. He titled his 1928 paper, "New Cancer Diagnosis." Later, he began working with a gynecologist named Dr. Herbert Traut, examining vaginal smears from female patients in the Cornell Hospital system. They published their now-famous book, "Diagnosis of Uterine Cancer by the Vaginal Smear," in 1943. Since that time, the Pap smear has become the most widely used and successful cancer screening test in the world. Over the past 50 to 60 years, the death rate from cervical cancer has dropped precipitously, mainly thanks to the Pap test.

While no woman looks forward to a pelvic examination, the Pap test itself is fairly straightforward. It should generally cause only minimal discomfort. With the patient's legs in stirrups, the doctor places a speculum into the vagina in order to see the cervix well, usually with the aid of a headlamp or speculum light. Then, the doctor places a thin plastic or wooden spatula against the cervix and sweeps in a circular fashion, also sampling any fluid at the top the vagina that may have pooled there. A thin brush is also placed into the cervical os (center opening) to obtain a slightly deeper sample of cells from that area. These samples are then placed onto microscope slides, which are sent to the laboratory and examined by a specially trained technician and/or computer. The evaluation of the specimens is supervised by a medical doctor called a pathologist, who's specially trained to determine whether cancer cells are present or absent. Most samples will be negative, some will contain definite cancer cells, while others will have cells that are indeterminate or suspicious and require further evaluation.

Since the Pap test has done an excellent job at decreasing the risk of deaths from cervical cancer, it remains the basic screening test. Most women (who haven't had cervical or uterine cancer) should follow ACS guidelines. Standard, conventional Pap tests should be performed annually, or the newer liquid-based Pap test may be performed once every two years.

The sensitivity and specificity of the two types of tests are similar in most studies. Women over 30 years old who've had three consecutive negative Pap tests may decrease the frequency to once every three years. Women over 70 years old may discontinue testing if they've had no abnormal tests in the past decade. Patients sometimes will ask about recommendations for their daughters also. Young women should begin screening three years after becoming sexually active or at age 21, whichever comes first.

For many years, doctors and scientists have known that certain strains of the human papillomavirus (HPV) cause most cases of cervical cancer. Scientists have now devised testing to detect the presence of HPV DNA in samples obtained in a similar method to the Pap test. Recently, major studies have shown that this HPV DNA testing improves the accuracy for detecting cervical intraepithelial neoplasia (CIN; abnormal, precancerous cells that require treatment to prevent cervical cancer). In light of these tests and the vaccines against HPV infection which are currently recommended for patients ages 9 to 26, the future of cervical cancer screening is likely heading for further changes. In fact, the ACS now already recommends that HPV testing be added to Pap for patients over 30 once every three years based on these studies.

Colorectal Cancer Screening with Colonoscopy

The ACS recommendations for colorectal cancer (CRC) screening are different than for other cancers in that they give doctors and patients multiple options. There are simple tests that just evaluate for the presence of cancer cells, and there are more complex and expensive tests that screen for both polyps (potentially precancerous growths) and cancer. In the former group, there's clear evidence that fecal occult blood testing decreases the death rate due to CRC among several large population studies that have been performed. This simple, low-cost test is an excellent option for screening, particularly in geographic regions or among populations where more elaborate testing isn't possible. Among the latter group of more elaborate tests, there are four choices.

Flexible sigmoidoscopy is a procedure during which the doctor, usually a gastroenterologist who specializes in diseases of the GI tract, places a scope into the anus to look at the last portion of the colon, called the rectosigmoid.

The remainder of the colon isn't inspected. Therefore, cancers that may be present in the upper/right portion of the colon may be missed with this test.

Colonoscopy is a similar procedure, usually performed by a gastroenterologist, which allows direct visualization of the lining of the entire colon. General surgeons as well as colorectal surgery specialists also perform colonoscopies. Patients are sedated, and the procedures are most frequently performed on an outpatient basis in roughly 30 minutes. Most people complain more about the colon cleansing preparation the day prior than they do about the procedure itself. Colonoscopy is the only procedure of the four options listed for screening both polyps and cancer during which the physician is able to directly see the entire surface of the bowel that's at risk for developing disease.

Double-contrast barium enemas still exist, much to the surprise and dismay of most people who've ever endured one of these procedures. They're performed in the department of radiology. The thick white barium is pumped through the anus into the colon, then x-ray pictures are taken. They're reviewed for possible abnormalities in the wall of the colon by the radiologist. While the test looks at the entire colon, it does so in the form of x-ray pictures rather than direct visualization of the lining of the bowel as with colonoscopy.

Lastly, CT or virtual colonoscopy is a more recently developed imaging study. Computed tomography (CT) images are obtained in such a fashion as to be able to reconstruct pictures of the entire colon. These studies can be very accurate at evaluating for the presence of cancer. However, in my opinion, given the relative safety of colonoscopy, which allows direct visualization of the bowel wall and any potential polyps or tumors, the indications for virtual colonoscopy are currently very limited.

So, while the ACS offers a choice among these four procedures, the first choice for CRC and polyp screening for the vast majority of the author's patients is colonoscopy. The data for its effectiveness is fairly strong. The standard recommendation for colonoscopy is a baseline study at age 50 to 55. Some studies indicate that most of the survival benefit is from this initial exam. Repeat examinations are required only once every 10 years for most patients who don't have suspicious polyps or invasive cancer.

PART II

CANCER TREATMENT OPTIONS FOR THE 20 MOST COMMON TYPES

Essentials of Cancer Diagnosis, Staging, and Treatment

Part II of this book outlines the basics of cancer treatment, staging, and diagnosis, presented alphabetically by disease site for convenient reference. The top 20 cancer types discussed herein account for over 90% of all cancers diagnosed in the United States each year. While the statistics quoted are from this country, the principles of cancer diagnosis, staging, and treatment apply to most of the developed world.

In order to personalize the medical information that's presented about cancer treatment in Part II, each chapter begins with an individual patient's story. These fictional patients are based upon thousands of real patients that the author has seen and treated over the past 14 years as a cancer specialist. The bulk of each chapter is spent describing how each of the common cancers is most frequently diagnosed and staged, followed by options for cancer treatment. Each chapter then concludes with the fictional patient's individual treatment plan and outcome. Hopefully these stories will bring home critical points about each cancer for the reader.

Since there are medical terms and procedures that occur repeatedly throughout this section of the book, they'll require review here. Some of the most important terms are in bold print below.

Cancer Statistics and Warning Signs

It's important to begin with an understanding of the magnitude of the problem at hand. Therefore, the description of each individual cancer type starts with the number of patients in the United States who are diagnosed each year, the death rate, as well as the lifetime risk of developing that particular cancer. Cure rates for each disease are reviewed, generally for both early and advanced stages.

Risk factors include actions, behaviors, exposures, and genetics that leave certain people more prone to develop a particular type of cancer. Symptoms are the complaints that patients bring to their doctors that may be warning signs of cancer. Signs are actual findings on physical examination by the patient's primary doctor or oncologist (cancer specialist) that may raise the suspicion for the presence of cancer.

Diagnosis

Cancer diagnosis is the process of determining whether a patient has cancer and, if so, what type. Most cancers are diagnosed by biopsy, the removal of some (or occasionally all) of the tissue from a mass or tumor. A biopsy may be performed by a surgeon, radiologist, or other medical specialist. Some primary care physicians even perform skin biopsies in their office. The biopsy tissue is then sent to a laboratory, where trained technologists cut the tissue into thin sections and prepare it to be reviewed by a medical specialist called a pathologist. The pathologist will view the tissue on a slide under a microscope. Special studies or stains may also be performed on the tissue to determine its type. The first decision that this physician must make is whether the tissue is malignant (cancer) or benign (not cancer). Next, if the tissue is found to be malignant, the pathologist must decide what type of cancer is present. The most common kind of cancer is called a carcinoma. The vast majority of cancers are this type. Lymphomas and sarcomas are two other types of solid tumors. Leukemia and myeloma are types of cancer that are sometimes called "liquid tumors" because the cancer cells in these diseases exist mainly in the blood and bone marrow.

Staging

Cancer staging refers to the process of determining whether the cancer is "early or late." Once a specific type of cancer has been diagnosed from a biopsy, oncologists then need to know whether the tumor is localized, whether it's spread to lymph nodes nearby, or whether it's metastasized (spread to distant sites), usually making the cancer incurable. This valuable information guides treatment recommendations.

The most common cancer staging system used by specialists in the United States is the American Joint Commission on Cancer (AJCC) Tumor Node Metastasis (TNM) staging system. It's revised and refined every few years based on advances in pathology and imaging that may affect staging and cure rates. It's currently in its seventh edition. All cancer specialists in the country have a copy of this book (or they should). Since the specific details of staging are beyond the scope of this guide, interested readers are referred to the *AJCC Cancer Staging Manual, Seventh Edition* in that regard. The clinical staging process is based on the oncologists' findings at the time of physical examination of the patient, the results of any pertinent imaging studies, as well as specific lab tests for some cancers. Common imaging tests that may be recommended for staging include:

X-rays—diagnostic radiation used to make basic pictures of the body; particularly helpful in evaluating bones for cancer involvement.

Ultrasound—high-frequency sound waves that are used to take pictures of the inside of the body.

CT (Computerized Tomography)—diagnostic imaging that combines multiple x-ray type images to show a patient's internal anatomy. CT scans may reveal whether a cancer is confined to the primary site (where the cancer started) or has spread to lymph nodes or other organs in the body. Patients are placed within a large circular tube that generally does *not* cause claustrophobic patients to become anxious.

MRI (Magnetic Resonance Imaging) —diagnostic imaging test that uses magnetic waves to create a detailed picture of a patient's internal anatomy. MRI scans may reveal whether a cancer is confined to the primary site, or has spread to lymph nodes or other organs in the body. Patients are placed within a small, circular tube that may cause claustrophobic patients to become anxious, so antianxiety medications are sometimes prescribed.

Mammography—imaging of the breast tissue that may be performed as a screening or diagnostic test.

Bone scan—diagnostic imaging of the skeleton to determine whether cancer has spread to bones.

PET (Positron Emission Tomography)/CT Scans—imaging study that combines anatomic information from CT scan with functional information from the PET scan, the latter of which shows areas in the body that are using glucose (blood sugar) at a more rapid rate than other tissues. Cancer cells tend to use glucose more rapidly than other cells, so areas of malignancy appear bright on these scans. Infection and inflammation may also appear bright on PET scans.

Treatment

Cancer treatment can be broadly broken down into main categories, including local, regional and systemic. The two most common types of local and regional treatments for cancer are surgery and radiation therapy. The most common type of systemic therapy is chemotherapy. However, multiple other exciting types of systemic treatment have been developed to combat and often cure cancer over the past couple of decades.

LOCAL AND REGIONAL TREATMENT

Surgery

The most widely known type of local anti-cancer treatment is surgery. Many types of cancer, if detected early enough, may be cured by surgical removal of the tumor mass or masses. In most major cancer centers and hospitals, specially trained surgeons called surgical oncologists will evaluate and operate on patients, depending upon the specific disease site. In general, the goal of cancer surgery is to remove the entire diseased area with negative surgical margins (rim of normal, noncancerous cells around the tumor when viewed under the microscope). Some cancers require wider margins of normal tissue to be removed around the tumor than others in order to minimize the risk of recurrence (relapse; cancer coming back). Many advances have occurred in the field of surgical oncology over the past 20 to 30 years. Surgical procedures which are unique to a specific cancer types will be discussed in each chapter.

Radiation Therapy

High-energy radiation treatment kills cancer cells. This type of anti-cancer treatment can be delivered on its own, before or after surgery, and with or without chemotherapy. Most commonly, radiation therapy (RT) is delivered by means of a high-tech, expensive machine called a linear accelerator. Usually the treatments are delivered in small daily doses called fractions, often over the course of several weeks. RT is delivered in these frequent small doses in order to minimize the risk of damage to normal tissues and cells, which are generally able to repair the RT injury over short time, while cancer cells usually cannot. The daily and total dose of RT is measured in **Gy** (pronounced "gray"; unit of absorbed radiation dose).

In 2010, the two most common types of RT used to treat cancer are three-dimensional conformal (3DCRT) **and intensity modulated (IMRT)**. 3DCRT is performed after obtaining imaging of the part of the patient's body that's affected by cancer, usually via CT scan. Then, an RT plan is created utilizing special computerized planning software. This plan usually incorporates multiple RT beams delivered to treat tumor target(s) outlined by a type of cancer specialist called a radiation oncologist, who will already have taken a thorough medical history and performed a physical examination of the patient. The RT targets may include not only grossly visible tumor but also areas of potential microscopic cancer spread, as well as a small margin for organ and patient movement during treatment. IMRT takes the 3DCRT process a step further by varying the intensity of each radiation beam, often by creating multiple smaller beams within each beam. IMRT often (but not always) allows the treating radiation oncologist to deliver a higher dose to the tumor target(s) while minimizing radiation dose to surrounding normal tissues when compared to 3DCRT. Image-guided radiation therapy (IGRT) is also frequently used to treat certain cancers, often in conjunction with IMRT. The IGRT process allows the treating RT technologist and supervising radiation oncologist to view the tumor or treatment site on a daily basis and make fine adjustments to patient position. It further ensures accurate RT delivery to the tumor target(s).

There are a few other special kinds of RT. Proton therapy is another type of RT that has excellent ability for focusing radiation dose, but is limited in its availability due to the expense of constructing these facilities. As of this writing, there exists no clear proven benefit for proton treatment over 3DCRT or IMRT in the treatment of common cancers in adult patients including prostate cancer. Stereotactic radiosurgery (SRS) is highly focused, high-dose RT for treatment of tumors in the brain. SRS can be delivered by means of several different types of expensive medical radiation machines. Usually this treatment is delivered in a single, high-dose fraction. However, fractionated SRS has a role in the treatment of certain brain tumors. Lastly, stereotactic body radiation therapy (SBRT) can be used to treat certain tumors in the body with high doses of highly focused RT delivered in a single or a few fractions. Common indications for SBRT include medically inoperable tumors of the lung, liver, and spine.

The effectiveness of RT to cure or palliate patients' symptoms and improve quality of life depends on the type and stage of cancer. Roughly 60% to 70% of patients seen in radiation oncology departments have potentially curable cancer, while the other 30% to 40% have incurable disease when they're seen for initial consultation. These patients may require palliation of pain or bleeding to improve their quality of life. Side effects or toxicities from RT vary widely depending upon the site of the body that's being treated. They will be discussed within each chapter by disease site.

SYSTEMIC TREATMENT

Chemotherapy

This group of medications, usually delivered intravenously (IV; by vein) or orally (PO; by mouth), has direct killing effects on cancer cells. Chemotherapy may be recommended as part of curative treatment and also for palliation of patients with incurable, metastatic cancer. Either a single drug or a combination of multiple medicines may be recommended. It may be delivered before or after surgery, and before, during, or after RT. When chemotherapy is delivered during the course of RT, the regimen is referred to as concurrent chemoRT. Many cancers are treated with concurrent chemoRT definitively (by itself, without surgery), resulting in high cure rates. ChemoRT may also be delivered either preoperatively or postoperatively. Since there are a multitude of chemotherapy agents that have proven effective in the treatment of various cancer types, the different agents and combinations as well as their potential side effects will be discussed within each chapter.

Hormonal Therapy

Some of the most common cancers, such as those of the breast and prostate, grow at least in part as a result of hormones acting at hormone receptors on cancer cells within the body. Growth of these cancer cells can often be halted or slowed dramatically with medicines that inhibit (block) action of hormones on these receptors. These agents may be delivered PO, IV, or subcutaneously (SQ; under the skin). They may be delivered before, during, or after RT or surgery. They can be extremely effective anticancer agents and can improve patients' survival significantly.

Immunotherapy

The body's own immune system is a powerful anti-cancer tool in many ways. In fact, it's theorized that the reason that more people aren't diagnosed with cancer at earlier ages is that the body's immune system is constantly monitoring for rogue cancer cells and eliminating them. It's only when the burden of cancer cells overcomes the immune system that malignant tumors are able to grow and potentially metastasize to other sites. Brilliant scientists have designed and continue to develop multiple types of immunotherapy. One type, therapeutic cancer vaccines, often confuses people. This type of immunotherapy actually treats cancer rather than preventing it. Using patients' own immune cells attached to other anti-cancer agents, the vaccine seeks and destroys cancer cells or tumor masses that already exist within the body.

Other Biologic Agents

There are now multiple classes of systemic anti-cancer therapies that don't fit neatly into any of the above classifications. Since most of these medications are designed with a specific site or receptor on the cancer cell where they act, they're often referred to as targeted therapies. Many of these new, exciting anti-cancer agents are being evaluated daily in clinical trials. In fact, by the time this book is published, there will undoubtedly be several new targeted therapies in use. Two examples that are currently being used to treat and often help cure patients are epidermal growth factor receptor (EGFR) and vascular endothelial growth factor (VEGF) inhibitors. These and other targeted agents will be discussed by disease site within each chapter.

CLINICAL TRIALS

In order to determine the best type of treatment for a particular disease or cancer type, physician scientists perform clinical research. The highest level of clinical research is called a randomized controlled trial (RCT). A prospective RCT begins with a hypothesis or theory about a medical treatment and moves forward to answer a specific clinical question. In cancer research, this type of clinical trial generally tests the current best treatment for a specific cancer type and/or stage (treatment A) against a new and potentially better cancer treatment (treatment B). This format is also referred to as a phase III clinical trial. Patients who agree to participate in this type of trial are randomly assigned to either current standard treatment A or new treatment B. Neither the patient nor the doctor gets to choose which treatment the patient receives. In this way, patient and physician bias can be minimized, such that the results of the trial will be more likely to apply to the larger population with that specific disease or cancer type.

For RCTs that evaluate cancer treatment, the new experimental treatment B may involve a change in surgical management, RT dose or delivery, a new chemotherapy drug, or other systemic treatment. RCTs are the main vehicles that drive clinical research forward toward improving cancer care, and closer toward the goal of eliminating cancer altogether. Within the discussion of treatment strategies in each chapter, the major RCTs that have changed the standard management for common cancers will be reviewed.

Sometimes, though, RCTs aren't feasible for certain types or stages of cancer, generally those that are less common in relative terms. In these situations, other types of medical research provide important information that can help to guide future treatment decisions. Nonrandomized, prospective (forward-looking) trials at single hospitals, as well as retrospective (looking backward in time) studies of groups of patients treated in a specific manner, are examples of these types of medical reports.

Lastly, sometimes multiple RCTs are performed to answer a question about cancer, but the results appear to be conflicting or weak. In these situations, researchers will sometimes perform a meta-analysis. This type of research study usually combines individual patient information from multiple RCTs to improve the statistical power to detect a difference. Quite often, meta-analysis may combine 10, 20, or more entire trials together and reanalyze results based on thousands of individual patients rather than hundreds.

BLADDER CANCER

Miles's Story

Miles was a 72-year-old man who had been a lifelong smoker and, as a result, he had developed chronic bronchitis. He was a well-respected auto mechanic whose knowledge and expertise were sought after by virtually everyone in his community, even well into his retirement. He recently noticed that his urine had appeared pink over the past week. On two episodes, he passed bright red blood in his urine. He had a long history with his local urologist, whom he had seen over the years for a benign enlarged prostate, so he went to him about this bleeding. The urologist performed a cystoscopy, a procedure that involves putting a thin fiberoptic scope through the penis and urethra and into the bladder. The cystoscopy revealed a 3 x 3 cm (1.5 x 1.5 inch) tumor over the right lateral wall of the bladder. Biopsy confirmed a transitional cell carcinoma, bladder cancer. (To be continued....)

In the United States, roughly 71,000 cases of bladder cancer are diagnosed and 14,000 patients die of the disease each year. It's much more commonly diagnosed in men (about 53,000 cases per year) than in women (18,000 cases per year). The median age at diagnosis is 73 years old, and it's rarely seen in patients younger than 35. Lifetime risk of developing bladder cancer is approximately 2.4%, or one in 40 people. According to the NCI's SEER database, the survival rate at five years after diagnosis for all stages combined is

79%. For patients with pre-invasive cancer (50% of all cases), the survival rate is 97% at five years. For patients with localized disease, the five-year survival is 73%. Survival for patients with spread to lymph nodes is 36%, and it's 6% for patients whose disease has spread to distant, metastatic sites in the body.

Risks and Causes

While the general public is frequently warned about tobacco smoking causing lung cancer, smoking dramatically increases the risk of developing many other cancers, including bladder cancer. Other risk factors include chemicals such as phenacetin and the chemotherapy drug cyclophosphamide. Bladder cancer diagnosis is sometimes correlated with working in the rubber and dye industries. However, many patients who develop bladder cancer have no known risk factors.

Signs and Symptoms

The classic symptom of bladder cancer is hematuria, painless blood in the urine. Occasionally, patients will present to their primary doctor with complaints of pelvic pain or difficulty with passing their urine.

Diagnosis

Patients who are seen by their primary physician with complaints of blood in the urine are generally referred to a urologist, a surgeon specializing in the care of the genitourinary (GU) tract. The urologist will directly inspect the bladder visually by cystoscopy, a procedure where a very thin fiberoptic scope is inserted through the genitalia and urethra into the bladder. Biopsy of any suspicious lesions is performed. The most common type of bladder cancer is called transitional cell carcinoma, which accounts for 90% of all cases. Squamous cell carcinoma is less common, and adenocarcinoma is rare.

Staging

In addition to a thorough physical exam and cystoscopy to inspect the bladder, most patients who are diagnosed with bladder cancer undergo CT scan of the abdomen and pelvis and a chest x-ray. Intravenous pyelogram (IVP), a procedure where dye is injected into the upper urinary tract, may be done to check that there's no cancer above the bladder, in the ureters or kidneys. The AJCC TNM system is used for bladder cancer staging. Pre-invasive cancer (carcinoma in situ) is the earliest type of bladder cancer and is very common. Advanced disease includes tumors that invade deeply into the bladder muscle, into nearby organs, or spread to lymph nodes in the pelvis. Bladder cancer occasionally metastasizes to other sites, such as the lungs.

Treatment

The treatment of early disease is initially surgery. The most common form of surgery is a transurethral removal of the bladder tumor (called a TURB or TURBT). Postoperatively, the installation of a medicine called BCG into the bladder may be recommended. BCG is a form of immuno-therapy that's very effective against superficial bladder cancer. Treatment with intravesical (within the bladder) BCG is generally delivered once per week for six weeks. Reasons for treatment with BCG include a tumor that's high grade (very aggressive-appearing cells when viewed by the pathologist under the microscope), has recurred multiple times, or is associated with pre-invasive cancer throughout a large area in the bladder. In a well-known study, the addition of BCG treatment improved patients' chances for survival with-out cancer returning at 10 years up to 75%, versus 55% with surgery alone. Other RCTs have shown that BCG is superior to chemotherapy in preventing tumors from returning.

Treatment of locally advanced bladder cancer frequently involves major sur-gery called a radical cystectomy in which the urologist removes the entire blad-der and part of the urethra, the urinary tube leading to the genitals. In male patients, the prostate is also removed, and that procedure is called a radical cystoprostatectomy. Female patients usually have their uterus, fallopian tubes, ovaries, and a portion of the vagina removed. A lymph node dissection may be performed at the time of surgery. Most commonly, after removal of the blad-der, the urologic surgeon will then use a portion of the small bowel to divert the patient's urine. Sometimes, a portion of the bowel is reconstructed to form a new bladder, referred to as an orthotopic neobladder. Radical cystectomy is a major surgery, but curative for but curative for the majority of patients who are in otherwise good health and able to tolerate it. Five-year survival rates for patients range from as high as 90% down to as low as 40%, the latter usually in patients with tumors that invade deeply through the muscle wall beyond the bladder. Fortunately, this situation isn't common. Side effects of this surgery include bleeding, infection, urinary incontinence (leakage), vitamin B12 deficiency, stone formation at the surgical staple line, and sexual problems.

An alternative bladder cancer treatment for patients who are either unable or unwilling to have the bladder surgically removed is organ preservation with concurrent chemoRT. Patients treated with chemoRT for bladder cancer are often not in excellent health, since many have been seen by a urologist who deemed them a poor surgical risk. However, in order to be a candidate for bladder preservation with concurrent chemoRT, patients should have a complete TURBT initially. They should also have good bladder function, a tumor that doesn't block off the flow of urine from the kidney (called hydronephrosis), and minimal pre-invasive cancer. The most common chemoRT regimen involves approximately seven weeks of daily RT with concurrent cisplatin chemotherapy. For these patients who are, again, generally in worse overall health than those who undergo cystectomy, the survival rate at five years following diagnosis is roughly 50%. Approximately 80% of these patients are able to retain a bladder with good function. A major study testing the role of up-front chemotherapy delivered prior to chemoRT showed no benefit over chemoRT alone.

Common side effects of pelvic RT acutely include irritation of the bladder causing frequent or uncomfortable urination, irritation of the bowels causing discomfort or diarrhea, and fatigue. These effects usually resolve over a few weeks. Long term, there's a risk of bladder scarring or fibrosis, which, in the worst-case scenario, requires removal of the bladder and had occurred historically in up to 20% of patients treated with chemoRT. However, a study of significant late side effects among patients treated on multiple Radiation Therapy Oncology Group (RTOG) trials in the late 1990s revealed only 6% for urinary and 2% for bowel problems. Severe side effects, such as a fistula, a hole between the bladder and bowel or other adjacent organs, are rare.

The most common concurrent chemotherapy delivered in the setting of organ preservation is cisplatin. Side effects acutely include nausea and vomiting (which are generally well controlled on current anti-nausea medications), poor appetite, decreased blood counts, and fatigue. Serious but less common side effects long term include damage to kidneys and nerves in the hands and feet, and hearing loss for high frequency sounds.

Patients who have metastatic bladder cancer (that's spread to distant sites in the body) are incurable in all but rare cases. Palliative chemotherapy may be recommended to improve their quality of life. Gemcitabine and cisplatin are the two most commonly used agents in this situation. This doublet was proven superior to a four-drug combination of methotrexate, vinblastine, doxorubicin, and cisplatin (called MVAC) which had been the long-standing, fairly toxic treatment in years past. Side effects of gemcitabine include decreased blood counts, nausea and vomiting, poor appetite, fatigue and flulike symptoms. Less commonly, patients may develop mouth sores, diarrhea, or dyspnea (shortness of breath).

Palliative RT may be offered to patients who have bleeding or pain. Usually RT in the palliative setting is delivered to a moderate dose over a short, two-to-four-week course. Therefore, side effects are usually limited to mild acute irritation during urination or bowel movements. Severe toxicity is uncommon.

Miles's Bladder Cancer Treatment and Outcome

Following the cystoscopy that revealed the bladder tumor, Miles underwent a CT scan of the pelvis which confirmed the mass but revealed no evidence of lymph node or other pelvic involvement grossly. Bone scan revealed no gross evidence of metastases to bones. His urologist recommended a radical cystoprostatectomy with construction of a neobladder, which Miles underwent, revealing tumor penetration into the superficial bladder muscle but no further. Several lymph nodes were removed from the pelvis, but they contained no cancer. He received no further treatment. Postoperatively, he had some pain which resolved over a couple of weeks. He has been seen regularly by his urologist for the past three years with no evidence of tumor recurrence. Miles has adjusted well to his neobladder and is pleased with his outcome.

BRAIN CANCER

This chapter will be broken into two main parts: brain metastases and primary brain tumors.

BRAIN METASTASES

Billy's Story

Billy was a 71-year-old commercial fisherman who lived life hard. He smoked two packs of cigarettes each day and drank a fifth of whiskey every two days. However, he was strong and motivated enough that he continued to work full time. He developed a cough that wouldn't go away. In addition, he'd been getting terrible headaches each morning that made it tough to get through his routine on the boat. He hated taking even aspirin, so when two of them every eight hours wasn't relieving his pain, he finally decided he'd better go to the local medical clinic. His examination revealed high blood pressure and crackling sounds in his right lung when his doctor listened with a stethoscope. Due to Billy's worrisome symptoms and his being a nearly lifelong smoker, the doctor on duty recommended a chest x-ray and CT scan of his head. The chest x-ray revealed a mass in the central right lung. CT of the brain revealed an abnormality in the back of the left part of the brain. CT of the chest confirmed a 3 cm mass in the right lung with two smaller masses in the left lung, each measuring less than 1 cm, all worrisome for cancer. The remainder of the brain was unremarkable. Billy was referred to a pulmonologist (lung disease specialist). He performed a bronchoscopy, a procedure that involves passing a thin fiber-optic scope down the trachea in order to visualize the bronchial tree in the central lungs. This procedure revealed a mass pushing on the outside of the right main bronchus (airway). Biopsy during the bronchoscopy revealed an adenocarcinoma, nonsmall-cell cancer of the lung. (To be continued....)

Oncologists place brain tumors into one of two general categories initially: metastases (spread from another site) or primary (started in the brain). Frequently patients will say that a relative of theirs died from brain cancer. More frequently than not, upon further questioning, it's determined that the family member actually had a different type of cancer which metastasized (spread) from another site to the brain. This fact shouldn't be shocking since there are about 170,000 brain metastases diagnosed each year in the United States versus about 20,000 primary brain tumors (exponentially less). Of patients who are diagnosed with brain metastases, roughly half present with single brain lesions. The most common primary tumor sites that spread to the brain are also some of the most common cancers overall: lung and breast. For most patients who develop brain metastases, this disease spread indicates that their initial cancer is now incurable. For a small subset of patients, however, long-term survival is possible. These patients tend to be younger, in better condition overall, with good control of their primary tumor, and/or with a solitary brain metastasis.

Risks and Causes

The predominant risk for a diagnosis of brain metastases is a pre-existing diagnosis of cancer. In addition to lung and breast cancers, melanoma and kidney cancer frequently may metastasize to the brain. Other primary cancers spread there less commonly.

Signs and Symptoms

Many patients with primary cancers from other sites are found to have tumors that have spread to the brain despite being asymptomatic (not having any symptoms). Quite often, brain metastases are found at the time of initial cancer staging. Patients whose brain lesions are found incidentally, when they are asymptomatic, tend to fare much better than those who come to the doctor complaining of neurologic problems. Most other patients present with symptoms that are dependent upon the location of the lesion(s) in the brain. Some with tumors near areas that control motor skills will have difficulty with the arms or legs. Others may have a headache that doesn't go away with pain relievers. Still others may present with a seizure or symptoms that resemble a stroke, including difficulty speaking or finding words. Any of these symptoms should prompt an immediate visit to the doctor or emergency room, depending upon severity.

Diagnosis

MRI of the brain is the standard imaging test to evaluate patients suspected of having brain metastases. CT of the brain with contrast may be performed in patients who are unable to have an MRI. Biopsy by a neurosurgeon (surgical specialist for diseases of the brain and spine) may be performed to ensure the cancer type and to differentiate between metastatic and primary brain tumors.

Treatment

Patients who are in reasonable medical condition and have a solitary brain lesion that's located in a place within the brain that can be removed should have maximal safe surgical resection. A couple of major RCTs have shown that patients who are in excellent condition, have a solitary brain metastasis, and are treated with surgical resection have improved survival over those that receive only whole brain radiation. An RCT of surgery with or without whole brain RT revealed that patients who receive postoperative RT to the whole brain have a lower chance of the cancer recurring in the brain, as well as a lower chance of dying form neurologic causes. Therefore, a common treatment for brain metastasis for patients who are in great shape is surgery to remove the gross tumor, followed by whole brain RT to kill residual microscopic cancer cells. Side effects of neurosurgical resection depend largely upon the site of the tumor that is being removed, but also include risk of infection and, rarely, the chance of death.

For those patients who are unable or unwilling to undergo brain surgery to remove their tumors, focal high-dose RT in the form of stereotactic radiosurgery (SRS) may be performed with excellent overall results. Many patients who aren't candidates for surgery are excellent candidates for SRS. Among patients with tumors 3 cm (about an inch) or less, over 90% will have their tumors controlled with SRS. Acute side effects of SRS include headache and fatigue. In about 1% to 2% of cases, patients may develop focal permanent neurologic injury as a result of brain necrosis, tissue death of the normal brain that's next to the tumor.

For most patients with more than two or three brain metastases, the standard treatment remains whole brain RT, generally over a two-to-three-week course. This treatment tends to improve patients' neurologic symptoms and quality of life and may improve their overall survival. Common acute side effects include hair loss, scalp irritation, and moderate fatigue. The most common long-term side effect is difficulty with short-term memory or complex thinking. In rare cases, patients may develop significant difficulty with their thought processes. Focal, severe brain necrosis from whole brain RT occurs very rarely since the dose is low to moderate.

Billy's Brain Metastasis Treatment and Outcome

Following Billy's bronchoscopy that revealed adenocarcinoma, he underwent a PET/CT which confirmed abnormal activity in the right central lung dominant mass, two other lung nodules, and a questionable, tiny lesion in the liver.

The PET/CT scan did not evaluate his brain. Because he had a single lesion in the brain that was causing him problems, his brain metastasis was managed first. Billy was started on a course of dexamethasone, which promptly helped his pain. He was seen by a neurosurgeon, who recommended surgical removal of the left occipital lobe metastasis. However, Billy wanted no part of surgery. He was seen by a radiation oncologist, who discussed the option of stereotactic radiosurgery (SRS) for the brain lesion. He discussed possible side effects of headache and rare chance of focal injury to the normal brain tissue. Billy liked this option much better and proceeded. He underwent the planning MRI and CT scans of the brain, followed by the single fraction SRS treatment on an outpatient basis in the radiation oncology department. He tolerated it with no side effects. (For discussion of the systemic management of Billy's lung cancer, please refer to "Billy's Story" in the chapter on lung cancer.) Following completion of his chemotherapy, Billy did well for almost a year, at which time he underwent a repeat CT scan of the chest and abdomen. This study revealed multiple new lesions in both lungs as well as three lesions in the liver, all of which were consistent with a recurrence of his cancer. A restaging brain MRI revealed no new lesions there. His medical oncologist recommended a second-line chemotherapy regimen, which kept his disease stable for another six months, at which time the nodules in the lungs began to grow rapidly. Billy was feeling quite fatigued. He and his family decided upon supportive care with help from the local hospice. Billy died at home with his daughter at his bedside one month later.

PRIMARY BRAIN TUMORS

Anne's Story

Anne was a 58-year-old woman with a history of high blood pressure and a few minor surgeries. She was otherwise in good health. In addition to her full-time job as an administrative assistant, she liked to garden and spend time with her family, including her two young grandchildren. One day, while she was preparing dinner for the family, her husband noticed that she seemed confused. She was having difficulty finding the correct words to answer his simple questions. In retrospect, she had also been having an increasing headache over the past one to two weeks. Because of these worrisome symptoms, Anne's husband drove her to the emergency department, where an examination confirmed expressive aphasia (difficulty speaking the words in her mind). A CT scan of the brain revealed what appeared to be a mass in the brain. MRI of the brain confirmed a 2.2 x 2 cm (about 1 x 1 inch) mass on the left side of the brain near an area that controls speech. Anne was seen by a neurosurgeon who recommended removal of the mass, which appeared to be malignant on the MRI scan. (To be continued....)

There are approximately 20,000 cases of primary brain tumors diagnosed in the United States each year, exponentially less than the number of brain metastases. The median age at diagnosis is about 55 years old.

Unfortunately, primary brain tumors are diagnosed in children through adulthood into old age. The lifetime risk of a primary brain tumor diagnosis is 0.6%, or about one in 166 people. While the overall five-year survival from the time of diagnosis is 35% according to the NCI's SEER statistics, cure rates vary significantly depending upon the primary tumor type. Most of the discussion in this section focuses on malignant brain tumors, as well as a very brief synopsis of a couple of the most common benign tumors.

Risks and Causes

Most patients don't have a specific known risk factor prior to being diagnosed with a brain tumor. The risk of developing a primary brain tumor is higher in older patients. Whites have a higher risk than other races, except for meningiomas, which occur more commonly in blacks. Less commonly, patients are found to have a familial or genetic abnormality that puts them at increased risk. Long-term cell phone usage remains under close scrutiny, but a definitive link to the development of brain tumors hasn't been shown.

Signs and Symptoms

The most common symptoms of primary brain tumors include headache, seizures, nausea, and vomiting, the latter of which is classically worse in the morning. Family or relatives may notice stroke-like signs, depending on the location of the tumor. Often slow onset of symptoms may indicate a less aggressive tumor, whereas rapid onset may indicate more aggressive cancer.

Diagnosis

As is the case with brain metastases, the standard imaging for primary brain tumors is MRI with gadolinium contrast. MRI shows brain anatomy, as well as presence of any small tumors, in better detail than CT. Occasionally, PET scanning may be obtained of the brain. Other special scans, including magnetic resonance spectroscopy (MRS), may be performed, though mainly at major academic research hospitals. For patients who have unresectable tumors, biopsy by a neurosurgeon is often feasible and may help to guide treatment recommendations. Otherwise, surgical resection of the tumor routinely yields the brain tumor diagnosis, following review of the tumor material by a pathologist.

Treatment

The most common malignant primary brain tumors are a group called gliomas. Treatment and outcomes for the few other common tumors, which are mainly benign, will be mentioned briefly.

GLIOMAS

In adults, the most common malignant primary brain tumors are gliomas. The most common type of glioma, also the most aggressive, is called glioblastoma multiforme (GBM) and accounts for roughly 30% of all primary brain tumors. The next most aggressive type of glioma, called anaplastic astrocytoma (AA), accounts for another 10%. Low-grade gliomas account for roughly another 10% of primary brain tumors.

Treatment

The standard initial treatment for most gliomas is maximal safe neurosurgical resection. Side effects of brain surgery for cancer depend largely upon the site of the tumor that's being removed, but also include risk of infection and rare chance of death. Postoperative treatment following surgery depends upon the type of glioma. Standard treatment for GBM includes RT delivered in daily fractions, five days per week, over a six- to seven-week course to a dose of approximately 60 Gy, with a concurrent chemotherapy drug called temozolomide. The RT may be delivered with standard 3DCRT or IMRT, depending upon several factors, including the patient's overall condition, the size and location of the tumor target in the brain, as well as its proximity to other critical normal structures, including the eyes and nerves. The most common long-term side effect of brain RT is difficulty with short-term memory and complex thinking. In rare cases, patients may develop permanent significant difficulty with their thought processes or memory. Focal severe injury, such as loss of vision or motor function due to necrosis (death) of normal brain tissue, may also occur rarely.

The addition of concurrent temozolomide to RT as postoperative treatment for patients with GBM was shown in a major RCT to improve overall survival compared to RT alone. Long-term follow-up revealed that about 10% of patients treated with chemoRT were alive five years later, versus only 2% of patients who received RT alone. A test can be performed on the tumor to see if it's likely to be responsive to the chemotherapy. Temozolomide is a chemotherapy capsule that's taken by mouth and generally very well tolerated. Side effects include headache, bowel irritation, fatigue, and, less commonly nausea and vomiting. Rarely, temozolomide may cause damage to the central nervous system. Many patients with low grade gliomas are followed closely with repeat MRI scanning, but receive no postoperative RT or chemotherapy. The median survival following diagnosis for patients with GBM for many years was 10 to 12 months, which has improved to about 15 months with temozolomide. Patients with AA have a median survival in the range of three to four years. These numbers don't mean that all patients will live for this duration. Rather, half of the patients will live longer and half will live less than the quoted times. An occasional patient with aggressive glioma is cured and lives for many years, though this situation unfortunately remains very much the exception.

Patients with low-grade gliomas have a much more favorable prognosis in general. There are differences in survival and outcome based on patient age, overall condition, tumor subtype, and tumor size. The role and appropriate dose of postoperative RT for patients with low-grade gliomas has been tested in RCTs. A major European trial revealed that patients receiving 54 Gy of RT over six weeks had a longer survival free of disease than those randomized to no postoperative RT. Two trials from the United States and Europe randomized patients to lower dose RT (45-50 Gy over five to five-and-a-half weeks) versus higher dose RT (59-64 Gy over six-and-a-half to seven-and-a-half weeks). Both trials revealed no benefit to the higher doses. In fact, one of the trials revealed worse survival with higher RT dose. Therefore, the standard postoperative course for most patients with low-grade gliomas incorporates 45-50 Gy RT. The side effects include acute partial hair loss, fatigue, and occasional headache. Patients may have difficulty with short-term memory chronically. The risk of severe or focal neurological injury is about 1% to 2%.

Anne's Primary Brain Tumor Treatment and Outcome

Anne underwent a craniotomy by her neurosurgeon who was able to grossly remove 95% of the gross tumor that was visible intraoperatively. Pathologic review of the specimen confirmed a glioblastoma multiforme (GBM), grade 4, with extension to the surgical margin in multiple areas. Postoperative MRI scan revealed persistent but significantly decreased abnormal enhancement in the area of the tumor when compared to her preoperative MRI. She was referred to a radiation oncologist, who recommended postoperative IMRT. Anne saw a medical oncologist, who recommended temozolomide to be delivered concurrently with her IMRT and for several months thereafter. She tolerated the chemoRT with expected fatigue and hair loss over the local area on her scalp. She had no nausea and minimal headache. Anne did well with no evidence of recurrence until 15 months following completion of her treatment, when a repeat MRI (which she had every 3 months) revealed abnormal enhancement with an associated mass adjacent to the prior tumor bed. Open biopsy confirmed a recurrence of her disease. She was enrolled on a clinical trial of a promising new therapy which kept her disease from progressing for another six months. At that time, she declined significantly. Anne, her family, and her medical team convened. They decided upon comfort care only, with support from the local hospice. She died at home with her husband and hospice nurse at her bedside six weeks later.

Meningiomas

Meningiomas account for roughly 20% of primary brain tumors and occur more commonly in women than men, by a ratio of roughly two to one. Only 10% of these primary brain tumors are malignant. While many of them are found incidentally at the time of MRI scanning of the brain for other reasons, the most common symptoms that patients may develop include headache and confusion. However, symptoms are largely dependent upon location of the tumor.

Although most meningiomas are benign, many require treatment due to their causing mass effect (pushing) on nearby normal brain tissue. Maximal safe neurosurgical resection is the standard of care to treat the vast majority of patients. Postoperative RT is generally reserved for patients who undergo less than complete resection or whose tumors are found to be atypical or malignant upon review by a pathologist. For most patients with benign meningiomas, the likelihood of being free from tumor progression five years after diagnosis is greater than 95%. On the other hand, those with malignant meningiomas have a less than 50% chance of being alive without tumor progression five years after treatment. Focal high-dose SRS may also be used to treat meningiomas. In one large series, more than 90% of patients required no further treatment and were pleased with their outcome. Side effects of postoperative RT are dependent upon tumor location and RT beam direction. They include fatigue, local hair loss, and long-term risk of worsened short-term memory or thinking ability. Focal severe brain or nerve injury due to necrosis may occur in 1% to 2% of patients.

Pituitary Adenomas

These benign tumors account for 10% to 15% of primary brain tumors. Roughly 75% are functional, meaning that they produce hormones, and the other 25% are nonfunctional. Functional adenomas may be treated with medications, depending on the type of hormone that they produce. However, the standard initial management for most pituitary tumors is surgery. In addition to the usual surgical risks of infection and bleeding, a permanent decrease in critical hormone levels may result, requiring lifelong replacement.

The risk of this condition called hypopituitarism is about 30% at diagnosis, another 20% postoperatively, and yet another 20% after postoperative RT if required. Usually, only those patients who are unable to have complete removal of their tumor require postoperative RT. Their chance of being alive without recurrence or progression of their tumor at ten years following diagnosis is about 90% overall.

Acoustic Neuromas

These benign tumors that arise near the ear canal make up about 5% of primary brain tumors. They develop from abnormal cells on nerve coverings. The main nerves that control hearing, as well as expression and sensation of the face can be involved. The median age at diagnosis is 40 years old for those that occur in the general population. Some people with an uncommon disease called neurofibromatosis type 2 develop acoustic neuromas at a median age of 20 years old. When patients have acoustic neuromas on both sides (bilateral), neurofibromatosis can be virtually assured. Standard treatment for acoustic neuromas is either surgery or RT. The RT may be either fractionated over a standard six-week course or SRS in a single fraction. It's thought that fractionation may decrease the risk of RT-related hearing loss in patients who still have good function. Maintaining the SRS dose at or below 13 Gy decreases the risk of hearing loss also. Local control of tumor without progression following surgery or either form of RT is greater than 90% in most reports. Useful hearing is preserved in about 75% of patients. Facial muscle function and sensation are preserved in more than 90% of patients.

BREAST CANCER

Pamela's Story

Pamela was a 62-year-old nurse who was in excellent health. She was extremely fit, exercising five days per week, for an hour each day. Her nutrition was excellent as well. She had no significant past medical history other than two minor surgeries. Her family history was unremarkable, specifically without any history of breast or ovarian cancer. Pam had normal mammograms every year since age 40 until this year. Her most recent mammogram had shown a 1 cm mass in the upper outer quadrant of her right breast, in the ten o'clock position, with associated microcalcifications, which were new since her mammogram one year prior. The radiologist who reviewed her mammogram films recommended that the mass be biopsied. She was referred to a general surgeon who specialized in the treatment of breast cancer. The surgeon performed a needle biopsy, which revealed an infiltrating ductal carcinoma, breast cancer. (To be continued....)

Cancer of the breast is the most common cancer diagnosed in women (other than nonmelanoma skin cancer). In the United States, it's estimated that in 2010 about 210,000 patients will be diagnosed and 40,000 will die of breast cancer. The median age for diagnosis is around 60 years old, and it is rare before age 35. A woman's lifetime risk of developing breast cancer is 12%, or one in 8 women. Breast cancer can occur in men, though male breast cancer accounts for only 1% of all cases. According to the most recent NCI's SEER Cancer Statistics Review, the five-year survival following a breast cancer diagnosis for all stages combined is 89%. If the disease is localized, then the five-year survival is 98%. Patients with regional spread to lymph nodes have a five-year survival rate of 84%. Those who are diagnosed with metastatic breast cancer (spread to distant sites in the body) have a survival rate of 23% at five years.

Risks and Causes

About 90% of breast cancers are sporadic, meaning that they didn't develop as a clear result of genetics or family history. On the other hand, there are women who develop breast cancer as a result of clear hereditary and genetic risk factors. These include patients who carry the BRCA1 gene, which puts them at high risk for both breast and ovarian cancer, anywhere from 50% to 80% lifetime. Patients who express the BRCA2 gene are also at increased risk for breast cancer, including men. Women with two first-degree relatives have an increased risk of about 13%. Genetic counseling is often recommended to patients and their families in these situations. Uncommon genetic syndromes that increase the risk of breast cancer include Cowden's, Li Fraumeni, and Muir syndromes.

It's clear that women with early menarche (beginning of menstruation or "periods"), late menopause ("change of life"), no breast feeding, and those who are nulliparous (have never been pregnant and delivered a child) are at increased risk. In addition, women with a benign problem of the breasts called atypical ductal hyperplasia have a relative risk of developing breast cancer that's at least five times higher than the general population. Patients with a history of having benign breast cysts removed have a relative risk of developing breast cancer that's three times that of the general population. Prior radiation exposure to the breast, particularly at a young age, also increases the risk of future breast cancer. A classic example would be a teenage girl who received RT as part of curative treatment for Hodgkin's lymphoma. She would be at significantly increased risk of developing breast cancer years later. Early mammographic and MRI screening is recommended for these patients.

Signs and Symptoms

Most women who have been diagnosed with breast cancer have it discovered when they're asymptomatic (have no symptoms). These cancers are most frequently diagnosed following an abnormal routine mammogram. When patients do notice abnormalities, the most common complaints are a painless mass in the breast or under the arm, dimpling or changing in the breast skin, or occasionally a diffusely red breast with thickening. The latter may be a sign of inflammatory breast cancer, a particularly aggressive type. However, most women who develop a red breast don't have cancer, but rather have an infection of the breast called mastitis.

Diagnosis

A breast cancer diagnosis is usually made after mammography, often accompanied by ultrasound. Controversy surrounds the recommendations for frequency of screening women with mammography for breast cancer. However, there's absolutely no doubt that the procedure can save lives by diagnosing breast cancer at early stages. The classic findings on mammogram that are suspicious for cancer are the presence of a mass or a group of microscopic calcifications within the tissue of the breast.

In order to confirm the presence of a cancer that's suspected on imaging studies, patients generally undergo a breast biopsy prior to definitive surgery. These biopsies are frequently performed under mammographic or ultrasound guidance. Overall, the majority of biopsies performed are benign. Upon pathologic review, of those patients who are found to have invasive breast cancer, about 80% are diagnosed with a type called infiltrating ductal carcinoma. Lobular carcinoma makes up about another 10% of breast cancers. Medullary, tubular, and other subtypes of invasive cancer are less common. Pre-invasive cancer called ductal carcinoma in situ (DCIS) is another very common diagnosis. Important pathologic information is gained at the time of breast biopsy, as well as at the time of definitive surgery, that helps to guide treatment. These critical factors include tumor size, grade, margin status (whether the surgeon was able to resect all of the tumor with a rim of normal tissue around it), hormone receptor status (the presence or absence of estrogen and progesterone receptors on the tumor cells), whether the HER2/neu gene is amplified and the HER2 protein is overexpressed in the tumor, as well as other molecular information about the biology of the cancer.

Staging

After a breast cancer diagnosis is made, surgeons at many hospitals are now ordering MRI of the affected breast, and occasionally the contralateral (other) breast for "local staging." However, this practice may be currently causing as much harm as good. It appears to be a situation where an expensive technology is assumed to be an improvement in medical care, although the data to support it are lacking. For instance, the medical literature shows that for every two new true cancerous lesions detected in the breast, MRI also detects one false lesion (not cancer). In a major RCT, women who were randomized to breast MRI before surgery underwent the same rate of re-excision (second surgeries) as those who didn't get MRI. In fact, women who receive preoperative MRI are more likely to undergo mastectomy rather than breast conservation. Unfortunately, while breast MRI may change surgical management (from lumpectomy to mastectomy, for instance), it hasn't been shown to improve patients' outcomes. The benefit for MRI to evaluate the contralateral breast (on the other side) is also questionable, since for every one true cancerous lesion found, MRI detects one false lesion. Flip a coin?! Wise surgeons who order breast MRIs evaluate them carefully with their radiology colleagues and biopsy suspicious lesions prior to submitting women to mastectomies. In summary, while there are clinical situations where breast MRI may be helpful, widespread use for screening and/or local staging of breast cancer preoperatively can't be recommended currently.

The main reason for breast cancer staging is to ensure there's no gross evidence of cancer outside the breast that would change treatment recommendations or prognosis. Breast cancer is clinically staged (based on information available prior to surgery) according to the AJCC TNM staging system. Pathologic breast cancer staging is then completed based on information gained after review of the surgical specimen(s). Pathologic stage should be recorded along with clinical stage, since it may alter recommendations for therapy significantly. Blood work usually includes complete blood count, serum chemistries, and liver function tests. Imaging may include CT scan of the chest, abdomen, and pelvis as well as a bone scan in patients with more advanced or aggressive disease. In recent years, PET/CT has replaced the combination of CT and bone scan at many major centers for staging. Patients with advanced disease and neurologic symptoms may also undergo brain MRI to evaluate for the presence of brain metastases.

Early stage patients are those with small tumors and no evidence of lymph node involvement. The most favorable tumors also are slow-growing (as measured by grade and several other biologic parameters), with positive hormone receptors. Patients with locally advanced disease include those who have large tumors, involvement of the breast skin or chest wall, and/or extensive lymph node involvement.

Patients with distant metastases are generally incurable. However, as opposed to many other types of metastatic cancer, breast cancer that's spread to distant sites in the body doesn't necessarily mean that the patient will die in the following months. In fact, many patients with metastatic breast cancer who respond well to systemic treatment may live for many years, often with a good to excellent quality of life. Factors that may influence the patient's overall prognosis include patient age and condition, tumor grade, surgical margins, hormone receptor status, HER2/neu overexpression, as well as multiple other new molecular, biologic factors that are being discovered on a regular basis.

While AJCC TNM staging allows cancer specialists to make treatment recommendations and broadly predict breast cancer survival rates for patients, it has limitations. For instance, some patients with stage I disease will develop local recurrences or distant metastases, while the majority of other women will be cured. Until recently, physicians had few insights into how or why certain patients' tumor biology was more aggressive than others. Over the past few years, however, understanding of breast cancer biology has improved significantly. Thanks in large part to advances in molecular biology, experts now categorize breast cancers into four different types: luminal-A, luminal-B, HER2+, and basal. Different treatment regimens are now being tailored to treat these different molecular subtypes. It's likely that dramatic advances and further changes will occur in this fashion over the next several years for the treatment of breast cancer as well as many other common cancer types.

Treatment

A simple classification of breast cancer treatment may be broken down into locoregional versus systemic. Most patients with breast cancer will require some form of both types of treatment.

Locoregional Treatment

The main two surgical options in the treatment of breast cancer are mastectomy, which is surgical removal of the breast, versus partial mastectomy (also called lumpectomy), which involves removal of the tumor mass with a margin of normal tissue around it. In the distant past, the vast majority of women underwent mastectomy. Historically, a radical mastectomy was performed which involved removal of not only the breast tissue and adjacent lymph nodes under the arm, but also a significant proportion of the chest musculature. Relative to modern surgical techniques, this procedure was very disfiguring. Over the past few decades, the standard mastectomy treatment, called a modified radical mastectomy, has involved removal of only the breast tissue and axillary lymph nodes. Specifically, this procedure leaves the pectoralis major chest muscle intact, making it much less disfiguring, and making plastic surgery reconstruction more feasible.

While some women may opt for mastectomy, the majority prefer breast conservation (BC). BC includes surgery, usually in the form of partial mastectomy, with or without evaluation of regional lymph nodes, followed by postoperative radiation therapy (RT). Most surgical oncologists who treat breast cancer routinely will perform a sentinel lymph node (SLN) biopsy at the time of breast surgery. This procedure involves injecting around the tumor or areola of the breast with blue dye and radioactive tracer which guides the surgeon to the first site(s) of lymph node drainage from the primary tumor. If these lymph nodes are removed and contain no cancer, then the likelihood of cancer cells being left behind in other lymph nodes is very low (less than 5%). On the other hand, if the SLN biopsy is positive for cancer cells, then the surgeon will usually perform a completion lymph node dissection (LND) to remove the remaining lymph node tissue in that region. In addition to removing more of the patient's tumor burden, the LND yields further diagnostic information that's often valuable in guiding treatment. The value of LND is mainly prognostic (to help patients and doctors predict risk of microscopic tumor cells possibly being present elsewhere in the body) rather than therapeutic, since RT can kill microscopic tumor cells in lymph nodes very well in most cases. Women with DCIS or pre-invasive cancer generally don't have lymph nodes evaluated since the risk of cancer cells spreading there is less than 1%.

Multiple major RCTs have shown that mastectomy is not superior to BC. These trials changed the standard of care for breast cancer surgery for most women over the past three decades. Many other RCTs which randomized groups of women between surgery alone versus surgery plus postoperative RT have revealed a significant decrease in the risk of breast cancer returning locally with the addition of RT. For women who receive partial mastectomy alone (no RT), the rate of breast cancer returning within the breast is approximately 3% per year. In patients who receive postoperative RT, that risk decreases to about 1% per year. When these major trials were analyzed in a meta-analysis (a big study that groups together patient outcomes from multiple trials), it was discovered that for every four local breast cancer recurrences that were prevented with postoperative RT, one woman's life was saved. The absolute benefit of postoperative RT tends to decrease in older women, particularly those over 70 and into their 80s. However, even in many studies of these older women, a small benefit may remain for postoperative RT in terms of decreasing the risk of breast cancer returning locally. In general, the benefits of RT after partial mastectomy are greatest for women who are in otherwise good health and have a low chance of dying from other major illnesses, such as severe heart or lung disease.

Standard RT in the setting of BC historically has been delivered in small daily doses or fractions, five days per week, over a six-week course. More recently, a couple of major RCTs revealed that for women with early stage disease (smaller tumors and negative lymph nodes), a shorter course of radiation over three to four weeks was just as effective and had fewer side effects than the standard six-week course of treatment. The common acute side effects of RT include irritation or redness of the skin, mild fatigue, low risk of pneumonitis (inflammation of the underlying lung), rare chance of rib fracture, permanent arm swelling, or significant firmness and/or chronic pain in the breast. There are only a few groups of patients who should definitely not undergo BC. They include women who are pregnant (because RT may harm the fetus), those with diffuse disease in the breast (because their risk of cancer recurrence in the breast would be too high), and those with multiple recurrences requiring multiple surgeries (because treatment would result in an unacceptable cosmetic outcome).

Patients who require or decide upon mastectomy for their locoregional treatment most commonly will not require postoperative RT. However, certain subsets of patients with more aggressive disease will need RT despite having mastectomy. These patients include those with very large tumors, positive surgical margins (where the surgeon was unable to remove the entire tumor with a rim of normal tissue around it), as well as those with multiple positive lymph nodes. Three major RCTs, one from Canada and two from Denmark, revealed a 10% overall survival benefit for postmastectomy RT for these groups of women. This benefit is actually huge in the realm of medical treatments, very similar to the survival benefit for breast cancer chemotherapy. In these trials, all patients were treated with mastectomy and systemic therapy (either chemotherapy or endocrine therapy), then half received RT while the other half did not. The results have been reported now with 20 years of follow-up for the Canadian trial, and there remains a 10% absolute overall survival benefit to women who received postmastectomy RT.

Patients who have pre-invasive breast cancer that lines only the ducts of the breast but doesn't invade the nearby tissue have a disease called ductal carcinoma in situ or DCIS. These women generally have the same locoregional treatment options as patients who have invasive disease: mastectomy versus BC. The main difference from invasive breast cancer is that DCIS rarely if ever is found in lymph nodes under the arm and it has an even higher cure rate. Only patients who relapse with invasive disease have a risk of dying from their cancer. The benefits of postoperative RT following partial mastectomy have been proven for the vast majority of these women in major RCTs. A couple of well-known but nonrandomized studies have suggested that in highly selected older patients with DCIS, radiation may be omitted with a low risk (about 1% annually) of pre-invasive or invasive cancer returning in the breast. Patients must have low to intermediate grade DCIS, with surgical margins that are widely negative after close pathologic scrutiny. However, to reiterate, the RCTs that have tested the role of postoperative RT in the treatment of DCIS following partial mastectomy (lumpectomy) have shown a clear benefit to RT, on the order of a 50% reduction in the risk of recurrent DCIS or invasive breast cancer.

Over roughly the past decade, a subset of patients opting for BC has been treated with accelerated partial breast irradiation (APBI). Because prior surgical studies of patients with breast cancer had shown that the vast majority of patients who relapsed in the breast after surgery did so at and around the surgical site (rather than elsewhere in the breast), surgeons and radiation oncologists decided to limit the area of RT to only that portion of the breast. The professional associations of surgeons and radiation oncologists that make guideline recommendations as to which patients should be offered APBI (off of a clinical trial) differ slightly in their opinions. However, there's general agreement that most women over 50 years of age with small tumors, favorable biology including negative lymph nodes, and negative surgical margins are good candidates for APBI.

Multiple nonrandomized studies now have shown that patients treated with APBI have a risk of the cancer returning in the breast of about 5% over five years. This result, 1% per year, is the same as standard RT to the whole breast. However, APBI has not been proven to be equivalent to (or better than) standard whole breast RT in a RCT. A major RCT is ongoing that randomizes patients to either standard whole breast RT or APBI by one of three different methods. Several thousand women have been enrolled and the results will be anxiously anticipated once the study closes. The obvious benefit to APBI is that it limits any potential side effects of RT to a small portion of the breast. At Coastal Carolina Radiation Oncology, the most common method of delivering APBI is via the MammoSite® Radiation Therapy System (Hologic, Inc.). As an added benefit, the treatment is delivered generally in high doses twice per day over one week rather than once daily over four to six weeks. The most common side effects of APBI are infection and seroma (firm fluid-filled area that can be tender) at the operative site or tumor bed in the breast. These can occur in about 10% of patients. Long term, there's a small risk of chronic pain and/or fibrosis (scarring) at the site. In rare cases, the surgical wound or incision site can fail to heal, requiring further surgery.

Systemic Treatment

Chemotherapy is the most well-known, and often feared, type of anti-cancer treatment that's used against breast cancer. Despite patients' anxieties, the vast majority of women who undergo chemotherapy for breast cancer tolerate it relatively well. It's generally recommended for patients with tumors greater than 1 cm, those with positive lymph nodes, and those with otherwise aggressive tumor biology. The latter group includes patients with tumors that are of the basal type (as mentioned above) or otherwise termed "triple negative," referring to lack of estrogen receptors, progesterone receptors, and HER2 protein overexpression on the breast cancer cells. This group of cancers tends to be much more biologically aggressive, with a higher risk for local and distant recurrence of disease, which can result in a higher risk of death. Specific systemic regimens are now tailored for these aggressive subtypes (discussed below).

Over the past several years, new genetic assays have been developed to help cancer specialists decide the best systemic treatment for patients, including who would most likely benefit from chemotherapy. These tests measure the levels of various important genes that may be present in tumor tissue. One of these is called the 21-gene Recurrence Score® assay, known popularly as the Oncotype DX test (Genomic Health, Inc.). This test was recently shown to be an independent predictor of which women will be at higher risk for their breast cancer returning in the locoregional area or metastasizing to distant sites in the body. The test results can affect medical oncologists' and patients' decisions and may also significantly decrease patient anxiety.

The most common chemotherapy drugs that are currently used for early stage breast cancer treatment in the United States are combinations of an anthracycline (doxorubicin, epirubicin), cyclophosphamide, and a taxane (paclitaxel, docetaxel). Several other chemotherapy options are available and active against breast cancer. The specific combination of drugs is chosen depending upon the individual biologic profile of the patient's tumor. Common side effects of these drugs include fatigue, poor appetite, decreased blood counts, hair loss, body aches, nausea, and a low risk of nerve injury in the hands and feet that is usually temporary. Rare but severe side effects include damage to the heart, nerves, and life-threatening infection. Most women receive four to six cycles of these medications, generally delivered once every three weeks. For women who are deemed chemotherapy candidates, the treatment usually begins a few weeks after surgery, prior to any planned RT.

Most patients whose tumors have estrogen and/or progesterone receptors benefit from endocrine therapy. In the treatment of breast cancer, the two most common classes of endocrine medications are selective estrogen receptor modulators (SERMs) and aromatase inhibitors (AIs). The SERMs bind to certain estrogen receptors but not others. They block some effects of estrogens (those that allow breast cancer cells to grow), while acting like estrogen in beneficial ways (such as improving heart health). Medications such as tamoxifen or raloxifene are examples of SERMs. Tamoxifen has been proven in RCTs to decrease recurrence of not only invasive, but also pre-invasive breast cancer (DCIS).

The AIs work differently. They inhibit or block the enzyme aromatase that converts androgen hormones into estrogen. Therefore, AIs allow less estrogen to get to the receptors on the cancer cells. Although they work by different methods, both have significant benefits to patients in terms of decreasing risk of local tumor recurrence as well as distant disease. Usually these pills are taken daily for five years after diagnosis, in order to decrease the risk of the cancer returning both locally in the breast and distantly in other parts of the body. In fact, they're sometimes even recommended preventatively for patients who don't have breast cancer but are at high risk for developing it. A recent meta-analysis (study that analyzed multiple trials together) revealed a slight benefit to AIs over tamoxifen, 3% less recurrences, for initial endocrine therapy as well as after two to three years of tamoxifen. Multiple RCTs have shown that most postmenopausal women with breast cancer that's positive for hormone receptors benefit from an AI during their postoperative treatment. The AI may be delivered as the only endocrine therapy, or may be given after completion of tamoxifen.

The most common acute side effects include fatigue, joint aches, and small amounts of weight gain. Patients taking tamoxifen have a small but real (less than one in 200) risk of developing a blood clot or uterine cancer. Cataracts may develop as well. AIs may have a negative impact on bone health. However, the benefits of these medications in dramatically decreasing the risk of breast cancer returning greatly outweigh the risks for the vast majority of patients with hormone-receptor positive disease.

Occasionally, surgical endocrine therapy is recommended for women who haven't yet gone through menopause. The most common surgery in that regard is called prophylactic oophorectomy, preventative removal of the ovaries. Since most estrogen is produced by the ovaries in premenopausal women, removing them significantly decreases the risk of future breast cancer in patients whose tumors are estrogen receptor positive. In fact, at least one study showed a clear benefit beyond tamoxifen for premenopausal women who had their ovaries removed.

The roughly 20% of patients with breast cancer whose tumors overexpress the HER2/neu protein benefit from yet another type of systemic treatment. The medicine trastuzumab is in a class of drugs called monoclonal antibodies (the "-mab" at the end of the word is the clue). It's a subtype of targeted therapy. The first major trials evaluating trastuzumab tested it in women with HER2+ metastatic breast cancer. Investigators in this RCT found that patients who received trastuzumab in addition to standard chemotherapy lived longer than those who received chemotherapy alone. Several other major RCTs have since been published that revealed a survival benefit to women with localized HER2+ breast cancer who received a year of treatment with trastuzumab, in addition to standard chemotherapy. Patients who opt for breast conservation may receive trastuzumab during their RT and continuing on thereafter for a full year. The main severe potential side effect of this medicine is a low risk of heart problems. The incidence of cardiac failure or death as a result of heart problems in the major trials was 2% to 4%.

Patients with metastatic breast cancer often develop painful or otherwise symptomatic sites of disease. A short course of palliative RT can improve their quality of life tremendously. For instance, the vast majority of patients who develop bone pain from metastatic cancer will have significant relief after palliative RT. Severe or chronic side effects are rare.

Lastly, some patients with breast cancer benefit from a class of drugs called bisphosphonates. They act by blocking the activity of cells that break down the bones, thereby strengthening the bones. Women with metastatic breast cancer that's spread to the bones are treated with bisphosphonates in order to decrease the risk of future fractures and other bony complications. RCTs have proven a clear benefit for patients with cancers that spread to bone including breast cancer, prostate cancer, and myeloma. These IV medicines are also used to treat patients who have dangerously high levels of calcium in their blood. They're usually delivered to patients on an outpatient basis like chemotherapy, once every few weeks, but over a much shorter time. Oral bisphosphonates, pills taken daily or weekly, are commonly prescribed to older women who don't have breast cancer, in order to treat osteoporosis. In 2010, a large case-control study involving more than 4,000 postmenopausal women revealed a protective effect for the oral medicines against the development of breast cancer. Perhaps a future RCT will provide a firm answer as to whether women should take bisphosphonates as a form of chemoprevention to decrease their risk.

Pamela's Breast Cancer Treatment and Outcome

After Pam's diagnosis by needle core biopsy, her breast surgeon discussed options of mastectomy versus breast conservation. She saw a plastic surgeon as well as a radiation oncologist. She opted for partial mastectomy followed by RT. Pam wanted to have accelerated partial breast irradiation (APBI), since she heard that the treatment only takes one week and a friend had a good experience with that type of treatment. However, she was felt to be a poor candidate by her surgeon and radiation oncologist due to the close proximity of the tumor to her skin, which would put her at extremely high risk of wound problems. She then underwent partial mastectomy, which revealed a 1.0 cm infiltrating ductal carcinoma, moderate grade, with negative surgical margins. Her tumor was moderately positive for estrogen receptors, but negative for progesterone receptors, negative for HER2/neu overexpression, and had a high proliferation (cancer cell growth) rate. A sentinel lymph node dissection revealed no evidence of cancer cells in three sentinel lymph nodes. Therefore, her pathologic stage was pT1bN0M0. Pam was seen in consultation by a medical oncologist, who recommended the 21-gene Recurrence Score assay of her tumor specimen to help determine whether she might benefit from chemotherapy. The test revealed that she was at high risk for tumor recurrence and would have a significant benefit from systemic chemotherapy. Pam underwent

---

four cycles of paclitaxel and cyclophosphamide IV chemotherapy in her medical oncologist's office which she tolerated relatively well. She had expected fatigue and hair loss, with mild nausea during treatment which was well controlled on anti-nausea medication. Pam then returned to her radiation oncologist and underwent a hypofractionated course of conformal RT to the whole breast over three-and-a-half weeks followed by a one-week radiation boost focused only on the tumor bed in the upper outer quadrant of her breast. She tolerated the RT well, with expected moderate redness of the breast which resolved by two weeks after completion of her treatment. Thereafter, she took tamoxifen for five years. Her doctor had discussed options of tamoxifen versus an aromatase inhibitor (AI), since the latter has been proven slightly more effective in decreasing the risk of breast cancer recurrence in patients who have already gone through menopause. However, the out-of-pocket cost of the AI was too high for her to afford on a monthly basis, so she opted for tamoxifen. Pam had mild joint aches and moderate hot flashes which were helped with vitamin E, but tolerated the medication otherwise fairly well. She has seen all three of her cancer doctors for follow-up care every three to six months over the past six years since completion of her treatment and has no evidence of cancer today. She is very happy with her cosmetic result after breast conservation. In fact, as a breast cancer survivor, Pam frequently speaks at her local community breast cancer support group in order to help patients who have been recently diagnosed.

COLORECTAL CANCER

Roberto's Story

Roberto was a 66-year-old Hispanic male who was still working as a chef at a four-star restaurant. He had a vivacious personality and an appetite for gourmet food. His past medical history included high blood pressure, high cholesterol, and adult-onset diabetes. He had never had a problem with his bowels and also never had a colonoscopy or other screening for colorectal cancer. When he developed rectal bleeding, he was very concerned, especially since he'd never had any problems with hemorrhoids in the past. He went to his primary doctor who performed a rectal exam. Although he couldn't feel any mass, he did perform a test on the stool specimen which confirmed the presence of blood. Roberto's doctor referred him to a gastroenterologist, who performed a colonoscopy. This procedure revealed a 7.5 x 5 cm mass in the sigmoid colon which was partially obstructing the bowel. Biopsy of the mass revealed an adenocarcinoma, colon cancer. (To be continued....)

Colorectal cancer (CRC) is one of the most common cancers in the United States. It's estimated to be diagnosed in 2010 in 143,000 patients, and 51,000 patients will die of the disease. The median age at diagnosis is 70 years old, and it's rarely diagnosed in people under age 35. The lifetime risk of developing CRC is about 5%, or one in 20 people. According to the most recent

NCI's SEER Cancer Statistics Review, the five-year survival following a colon cancer diagnosis, relative to the general population, for all stages combined is 65%. If the disease is localized, then the five-year survival is 90%. Patients with regional spread to lymph nodes or distant spread have five-year survival rates of 70% and 11%, respectively.

Risk and Causes

The vast majority of patients who are diagnosed with CRC don't have a family history of the disease or any particular genetic syndrome. Patients who eat a diet that's high in fat and low in fiber are at higher risk. There are a few inherited genetic syndromes that place patients at very high risk for developing CRC. Familial Adenomatous Polyposis (FAP) is a disease that's characterized by multiple aggressive polyps throughout the colon, and results in essentially 100% risk of developing CRC, usually by age 40. Gardner's syndrome and Hereditary Non-polyposis Colorectal Cancer syndrome are both also associated with a significant risk of developing CRC. Genetic counseling is generally offered to these patients and their families. In some cases, including virtually all patients with FAP, total colectomy (surgical removal of the entire colon) is recommended to prevent CRC.

Signs & Symptoms

The majority of patients diagnosed with CRC initially present to medical attention with complaints of bleeding or pain. Some patients complain to their doctors of general fatigue or tiredness and are found to be anemic, due to slow, long-term blood loss into the bowel which sometimes can't be seen in the stool. The symptoms of colon cancer may depend on the location of the primary tumor within the specific area of the colon. Patients who have locally advanced disease at the outset may complain of pain with bowel movements or difficulty passing their stools due to mechanical obstruction by the tumor.

Diagnosis

A gastroenterologist (medical GI specialist) or surgeon usually will perform a colonoscopy in order to visualize the entire colon directly. After giving medicine to sedate the patient, the GI specialist or surgeon inserts a thin, flexible fiberoptic scope through the anus into the rectum. Ideally, the entire lining of the colon is inspected. Biopsy of any suspicious lesions, masses, or polyps is performed during this procedure. Most CRCs are adenocarcinomas. Other types of cancer in the colon or rectum are rare.

Staging

The AJCC TNM system is used for colorectal cancer staging. Standard laboratory evaluation includes a complete blood count, chemistries including liver function tests, and a carcinoembryonic antigen (CEA) level. CEA is a marker in the blood that may be used to determine whether CRC has spread distantly and may be incurable. Imaging should include CT or PET/CT scans. Most major academic and larger community cancer centers also offer endoscopic ultrasound (EUS) for cancers in the rectum which evaluates the depth of primary tumor penetration into or through the bowel wall, and allows visualization of any enlarged nearby lymph nodes. Results of the EUS may guide preoperative or postoperative treatment.

In addition to cancer stage, other factors can predict outcome for patients with CRC. These include serum CEA level, presence or absence of multiple tumor deposits or invasion of nearby nerves, tumor response following preoperative chemoRT, and status of the surgical margin (edge of where the surgeon removed tumor). There are also several molecular factors that include the presence or absence of microsatellite instability (MSI) and/or a mutated K-ras gene.

Treatment

Patients with early stage colon cancer that's limited to the bowel wall usually have surgery to remove a portion of their colon, with an approximately 90% chance for cure. Locally advanced disease consists of tumors that invade through the bowel wall and/or into adjacent organs, or those with lymph nodes involved. These patients generally benefit from postoperative chemotherapy. A common regimen consists of a combination of three drugs called FOLFOX: fluorouracil, leucovorin, and oxaliplatin. Another popular three-drug regimen substitutes irinotecan in place of oxaliplatin and is known by the acronym FOLFIRI. The most common acute side effects include fatigue, diarrhea, generalized aches, and decreased blood counts. Less common severe side effects that may occur after treatment include chronic long-lasting numbness or pain in the hands and feet. Survival rates at five years after diagnosis range from 70% for stage II, down to 10% for patients with distant metastases.

Tumors that arise from the rectum have an increased risk of returning locally compared to tumors that begin higher up in the colon. The anatomic location of the rectum, low and deep within the pelvis, can make it challenging even for experienced colorectal surgeons to remove cancers with widely negative surgical margins. Tumors that are located at least a couple of inches above the anal sphincter are usually able to be removed (quite often after preoperative chemoRT) without need for a colostomy. The colorectal surgeon will perform a type of surgery called a total mesorectal excision, which involves removal of the rectal tumor with surrounding tissue and nearby lymph nodes all together in one sharply dissected specimen. The colon is joined to the anus, as long as the tumor can be removed with negative surgical margins, while leaving the anal sphincter muscle functioning. When tumors arise in the very low rectum, sometimes surgery requires creation of a colostomy. The bottom portion of the rectum and the anus are removed in this procedure, called an abdominoperineal resection. Most major cancer centers have support groups for patients who require a colostomy.

Standard treatment for patients with locally advanced rectal cancer generally incorporates both radiation therapy (RT) and chemotherapy. RCTs have shown an improvement in local tumor control as well as survival for patients randomized to RT (either preoperatively or postoperatively) over surgery alone. Other RCTs revealed that concurrent chemoRT was superior to RT alone. Either fluorouracil or capecitabine are most frequently used concurrently with RT, since FOLFOX and other more aggressive regimens would likely prove too toxic when delivered at the same time. Over the past couple of years, two RCTs have confirmed a benefit to preoperative rather than postoperative chemoRT. While the risk of cancer returning in the pelvis was low with both preop and postop chemoRT, preop treatment had fewer side effects. Preoperative chemoRT is the standard of care for locally advanced rectal cancer at most major cancer treatment centers.

The most frequent acute side effects of RT to the pelvis include irritation of bladder and bowel, causing frequency and/or discomfort with urination or bowel movements. Fatigue, poor appetite, and decreased blood counts are also common side effects of chemoRT in this setting. Rare long-term problems that pelvic RT may cause include permanent bowel or bladder injury requiring surgery to repair. Sexual dysfunction is not uncommon.

The most common chemotherapy drugs given during chemoRT for rectal cancer are either a continuous IV infusion of 5FU or the oral pill capecitabine, which is very similar in action to 5FU. The most likely side effects of these medicines are fatigue, diarrhea, and irritation of the lining of the mouth. A rare but sometimes severe side effect of these medicines is severe scaling of the hands and feet (called hand-foot syndrome). Even more rarely, patients may develop significant heart damage including potential heart attack with 5FU.

For patients with metastatic CRC, there have been a number of major advances to improve both quantity and quality of life. In addition to the chemotherapy regimens already mentioned, several other new, effective systemic agents have become available to combat CRC over the past decade. One example is bevacizumab which is in the class of drugs known as vascular endothelial growth factor (VEGF) inhibitors. These medicines block abnormal blood vessel growth, thereby normalizing the blood vessels around the tumor. Neovasculature, new blood vessels formed by the tumor in order to sustain itself, may shrink away dramatically after treatment with bevacizumab. Another type of targeted therapy is the class of drugs that blocks the epidermal growth factor receptor (EGFR) on tumor cells. The IV medication cetuximab is an example of an EGFR inhibitor that improves tumor cell kill when used in combination with chemotherapy against CRC.

The most frequent site of colon cancer metastasis is the liver. In fact, over 50,000 patients per year in the United States have liver metastases from CRC. Most patients with incurable CRC receive systemic chemotherapy. However, occasionally patients may undergo aggressive treatment with surgery, if they are in very good condition and have technically resectable liver metastases. Recent improvements in preoperative imaging such as MRI and PET/CT allow better selection of patients for surgery. Also, the ability of surgeons to look into the abdomen with a laparoscope preoperatively has spared many patients surgery that might not benefit from it. Patients who've had a long interval since their initial colon cancer diagnosis, who have fewer and smaller tumors in the liver, and who have the tumors removed with negative surgical margins tend to have the best chance of long-term survival. Improvements to minimize the side effects of surgery have also helped patients. A recently reported multi-institutional experience with "minimally invasive" liver resections (including laparoscopic surgery with or without "hand assistance") resulted in a five-year survival of 50% with no perioperative deaths among 109 patients. Lastly, it's now also common practice for patients to receive chemotherapy before surgery. At least one major European RCT revealed an improvement for patients randomized to FOLFOX chemotherapy both before and after liver resection, compared to the group that had surgery without chemotherapy.

In addition to open surgery, other local treatment options for treatment of liver metastases include radiofrequency ablation (RFA), radioembolization, and stereotactic body radiation therapy (SBRT). RFA uses alternating electrical current through multiple electrodes placed within tumors to destroy the tissue. Five-year survival rates for patients with liver metastases treated with RFA vary widely from about 15% to 55%. However, three of the largest series in the medical literature reveal a local recurrence rate of 7% to 14% and five-year survival ranging from 17% to 31%. These rates appear inferior to surgical resection, though these patients may be in worse shape at baseline compared to patients who are deemed medically fit for major liver surgery. Radioembolization involves delivery of localized radiation in the form of tiny spheres into the arteries of the liver. It's sometimes recommended for patients with more extensive liver metastases from CRC. A recent RCT revealed that radioembolization with 5FU chemotherapy was superior to 5FU alone in delaying the progression of cancer in the liver. Finally, SBRT is highly focused, high-dose external beam RT that's usually delivered in three to five fractions. It's been used most extensively for treatment of lung cancers in patients that aren't candidates for surgery with excellent results. However, some major cancer centers have been using this non-invasive technique to treat patients with liver metastases from CRC. Early results appear promising.

Roberto's Colon Cancer Treatment and Outcome

Following his positive biopsy at colonoscopy, Roberto was sent for a CT scan of the pelvis which confirmed the mass in his colon with no enlarged lymph nodes. However, two lesions in the left lobe of the liver were suspicious for cancer. Because the mass in the colon appeared to be nearly obstructing the passage of stool, his colorectal surgeon performed a resection of that portion of the colon. The pathologic review revealed a 9 x 5 cm adenocarcinoma with negative margins in all directions, but microscopic involvement with tumor cells in nine out of 14 lymph nodes. He also underwent resection of the two liver lesions by a hepatobiliary (liver, pancreas and bile duct) surgeon. This resection confirmed cancer in the two liver lesions, again with negative surgical margins. Roberto was seen by a medical oncologist, who recommended postoperative FOLFOX chemotherapy. He was not a candidate for bevacizumab treatment due to a history of a bleeding problem. He developed neuropathy (numbness) in his hands and feet near completion of the sixth cycle of chemotherapy and had significant fatigue throughout his treatments. Follow-up examinations and restaging CT scans revealed no evidence of disease recurrence until three years after completion of his chemotherapy. At that time, there was evidence of multiple small nodules in both lungs as well as two new large tumors in his liver. CT-guided needle biopsy of one of the liver lesions confirmed that his cancer had returned. His medical oncologist recommended enrollment in a clinical trial testing a promising new medication against the standard current treatment for recurrent colorectal cancer. Roberto agreed and was randomized to receive the standard second line chemotherapy, which he tolerated quite well. His disease did not grow for eight months.

Thereafter, however, the nodules in the lungs grew significantly. He and his family decided against further treatment. He received supportive care with hospice. He died at the local hospice care center six weeks later.

ESOPHAGEAL CANCER

Jimmy's Story

Jimmy was a 64-year-old construction foreman who saw his primary physician only on rare occasions, usually when a bad "cold" would keep him out of work. His past medical history was significant only for chronic gastroesophageal reflux disease (GERD). He never smoked and drank only a couple of beers on weekend nights. He and his wife loved to golf, which they were both looking forward to after his retirement the following year. Jimmy began noticing that foods like steak and chicken were causing him some discomfort when he ate them. On a couple of occasions, he felt like the food would get stuck in the lower part of his throat. When he went to see his doctor, he pointed to the middle of his chest, below the lower part of his breastbone. Although his physical examination was unremarkable, his doctor referred him to a GI specialist since his symptoms were continuing, despite Jimmy being on medicine to control his GERD. The GI doctor performed an esophagogastroduodenoscopy (EGD), placement of a thin fiberoptic scope through the nose to look directly at the lining of the upper GI tract (after sedation). He discovered an ulcer in the distal esophagus, near the junction with the stomach, which extended over an 8 cm length. Biopsy of the area revealed adenocarcinoma, esophageal cancer. (To be continued....)

Cancer of the esophagus and gastroesophageal or GE junction (area where the esophagus joins the stomach) will be diagnosed in about 17,000 patients in 2010 in the United States, while 14,500 patients will die of this disease. Rarely diagnosed prior to age 35, the median age for diagnosis is 68 years old. The lifetime risk of developing cancer of the esophagus is 0.5%, or one in 200 people. According to the most recent NCI's SEER Cancer Statistics Review, the five year survival following an esophageal cancer diagnosis for all stages combined is 17%. If the disease is localized, then the five-year survival is 37%. Patients with regional spread to lymph nodes and metastatic esophageal cancer have five-year survival rates of 19% and 3%, respectively.

Historically, esophageal cancer was much more common in men than women and more common in blacks than whites. In more recent years, however, adenocarcinoma has overtaken squamous cell carcinoma (SCC) as the leading type of esophageal cancer. White males are diagnosed with esophageal adenocarcinoma more commonly than others.

Risks and Causes

Patients who smoke tobacco, drink alcohol heavily, and eat or drink spicy or very hot foods or beverages put themselves at increased risk for SCC of the esophagus. This type of cancer tends to arise in the setting of chronic irritation. The upper esophagus is basically an extension of the throat. Most cancers of the head and neck are SCC, as are most cancers of the upper two-thirds of the esophagus. On the other hand, cancers of the lower esophagus and GE junction tend to arise in the setting of GERD, chronic reflux of stomach contents and acid. A condition called Barrett's esophagus that can result from chronic GERD is a clear risk factor for developing adenocarcinomas of the lower esophagus and GE junction.

Signs and Symptoms

The development of a tumor mass within the esophagus classically causes dysphagia (sticking sensation when swallowing) and/or odynophagia (pain when swallowing). Many patients have these symptoms when swallowing solid foods, but some may progress to have symptoms even when drinking liquids. Other patients with smaller tumors may have more mild symptoms, such as belching or reflux due to backflow of the gastric contents into the lower esophagus. On occasion, patients with more advanced disease may not notice any local symptoms of esophageal cancer but experience only weight loss, either unexplained or due to anorexia.

Diagnosis

Since chronic GERD is extremely common, a large proportion of the adult U.S. population is currently on various medications to deal with these symptoms. The vast majority, fortunately, will never develop cancer of the esophagus or GE junction. However, if GERD symptoms persist or are severe despite medications, then referral to a GI specialist is a good idea. Patients who have dysphagia or odynophagia for any reason should also be referred. The GI specialist may perform an EGD for direct visualization of the esophagus, stomach, and initial portion of the small bowel. Biopsy of any suspicious areas is usually performed during this procedure.

Historically, the most common type of esophageal cancer was SCC, occurring in the upper to mid esophagus, mainly in patients who use tobacco products or alcohol chronically. However, over the past 20 years, adenocarcinoma of the distal esophagus and GE junction has become much more common as a result of patients with chronic GERD. Only a small subset of these patients will develop cancer.

Staging

The AJCC TNM system is utilized for GE junction and esophageal cancer staging. Standard laboratory evaluation will include complete blood count and serum chemistries testing kidney and liver function. Imaging generally includes CT scan of the chest and abdomen, and PET/CT if available. Baseline PET/CT prior to treatment has been shown to be predictive of patients' outcomes. In patients who receive chemoRT prior to surgery, restaging PET/CT can predict the response to treatment as well as survival. Endoscopic ultrasound (EUS) can also be a useful baseline imaging study to look at regional lymph nodes. It's performed by a GI specialist and provides valuable information that may not appear on CT or PET/CT scan. In at least one study, EUS was just as accurate as a surgeon looking directly into the abdomen to evaluate nearby lymph nodes for the possibility of cancer. Bronchoscopy, placement of a thin fiberoptic scope through the trachea (windpipe) into the major bronchi (airways) of both lungs, may be recommended for patients with tumors in the upper esophagus, in order to ensure that they don't contain tumor.

Early stage cancer means tumors that are limited to the inner lining of the esophagus. Locally advanced disease includes tumors that extend through the wall of the esophagus and potentially into adjacent organs, as well as those with cancerous lymph nodes. Frequent distant sites of metastases include lungs, liver, and elsewhere in the abdomen. PET/CT staging is often useful in detecting sites of metastatic esophageal cancer that aren't visible on other imaging studies.

Treatment

Although early-stage esophageal cancer is uncommon, the standard treatment is surgery, either esophagectomy or esophagogastrectomy. The two most common procedures are called transhiatal and Ivor-Lewis esophagogastrectomies. The former involves resection through incisions in the abdomen and neck, whereas the latter incorporates an incision through the right chest. Both of these procedures are major surgeries. The most common potentially lethal postoperative complication of both surgeries is pneumonia, associated with a 20% risk of death.

The vast majority of patients with esophageal cancer will be diagnosed with locally advanced or metastatic disease. Those with locally advanced disease who are in excellent condition may be treated in several ways. However, the most common treatment for patients with locally advanced adenocarcinomas of the distal esophagus or GE junction in many major medical centers involves preoperative concurrent chemoRT delivered over an approximately six-week course, followed by a several-week break, then surgery (as described above). This trimodality therapy gives patients with locally advanced disease a reasonable chance for cure. Roughly 15% to 20% of patients who undergo preoperative chemoRT are found at the time of surgery to have no residual living cancer cells, when the pathologist looks at the surgical specimen under the microscope. This favorable situation is called a pathologic complete response (pCR). Again, PET/CT scan performed between chemoRT and surgery can often predict the response as well as long-term survival. Patients who get a pCR after chemoRT have a better chance for long-term survival than those who have residual disease at the time of surgery.

The preoperative chemoRT course can be difficult for patients to tolerate. The radiation is generally delivered using 3DCRT to a dose of about 50 Gy over a five-and-a-half-week course, in small daily fractions, five days per week. Acute side effects may include fatigue, bowel irritation including nausea, sore throat, and diarrhea. Severe late side effects such as a bowel obstruction or fistula (hole between the esophagus and breathing tube) are rare. The most common concurrent chemotherapy medications that have been tested in RCTs are cisplatin and fluorouracil. Acute side effects include nausea, fatigue, poor appetite, bowel irritation including diarrhea, and rare chance of severe peeling of skin from hands and feet (hand-foot syndrome). Rare but serious late effects include high-frequency hearing loss or permanent nerve damage.

Patients with metastatic esophageal cancer are generally treated with palliative chemotherapy to improve quality of life. Cisplatin and fluorouracil are again often used. Other medications that medical oncologists may recommend in this palliative setting which have activity against esophageal cancer include carboplatin, paclitaxel, docetaxel, and irinotecan. Occasionally mechanical stenting may be performed by a GI specialist or surgeon in order to keep the esophagus open and maintain nutrition if a large tumor is partially blocking it. Alternatively, or in addition, a short course of palliative RT may be recommended in order to help patients eat with less difficulty and improve their overall quality of life.

Jimmy's Esophageal Cancer Treatment and Outcome

Following his diagnosis, Jimmy underwent a staging PET/CT scan, which revealed abnormal activity in the distal esophagus into the top of the stomach, but no other abnormalities. His GI specialist performed an EUS which revealed that the

---

tumor extended through the entire wall of the esophagus. However, there were no enlarged nearby lymph nodes. His clinical stage was T3N0M0. A multidisciplinary conference was held among the various cancer specialists. They recommended preoperative chemoRT followed by surgical resection of the tumor. Jimmy tolerated the five-and-a-half weeks of conformal RT with concurrent chemotherapy with surprisingly little toxicity. He had moderate fatigue but no nausea, vomiting, or bowel irritation. Then he underwent a transhiatal esophagectomy, which revealed no evidence of residual tumor, only necrotic (dead) cells at the site of the primary esophageal mass. Multiple lymph nodes nearby were negative. After four years of follow-up, alternating visits with his multiple cancer doctors every three to six months, he is alive without any evidence of disease recurrence.

HEAD AND NECK CANCER

Clarence's Story

Clarence was a 57-year-old divorced bartender who had smoked a pack of cigarettes every day since he was 15 years old. On stressful days, he would smoke almost two packs. He drank a few beers and a shot or two of whiskey at the end of the night at the bar with his customers frequently. Clarence hadn't been to the doctor in over 10 years. When he developed a sore throat, he first attributed it to the flu. However, when it got worse instead of better over a month, he made a visit to the local medical clinic. The physician at the clinic felt a 2 cm lump in the left side of Clarence's neck at the angle of his jaw. He couldn't see any mass in his throat, but referred him to an otolaryngologist (ENT; ears, nose, and throat specialist). That doctor performed an examination with a mirror into the back of his throat which revealed a 5 cm mass in the base of his tongue. He also felt the enlarged lymph node in his left neck, biopsy of which confirmed squamous cell carcinoma, head and neck cancer. (To be continued....)

In the United States in 2010, it's estimated that about 37,000 patients will be diagnosed with cancers of the mouth and throat, and 8,000 patients will die of their disease. Cancers of the head and neck are diagnosed more than twice as often in men (25,000 cases per year) as in women (12,000 cases per year). The lifetime risk of a head and neck cancer diagnosis is about 1%, or one in 100 people. There are multiple different subsites that are all considered parts of the head and neck region. The main parts where the most common cancers occur are the oral cavity (mouth), oropharynx (upper throat), larynx (voicebox), hypopharynx (lower throat), and nasopharynx (area behind the nose and in front of the brain). Less commonly, cancers can occur in the head and neck glands, including the parotid (around the ear), submandibular (below the jaw), and minor salivary (along the roof of the mouth). Cancers also rarely occur in the nasal cavity and sinuses.

According to the most recent NCI's SEER Cancer Statistics Review, the five-year survival following a diagnosis of pharyngeal cancers (cancers of the throat, excluding the voicebox) for all stages combined is 61%. If the disease is localized, then the five-year survival is 83%. Patients with regional spread to lymph nodes and metastatic head and neck cancer have five-year survival rates of 54% and 32%, respectively. The corresponding five-year survival numbers for patients with larynx (voicebox) cancer are 61% overall, 78% if localized, 42% if regional and 33% if distant metastases.

Risks and Causes

The leading risk factor for the development of squamous cell cancers of the head and neck (HNSCC) is chronic use of tobacco products, most frequently smoking cigarettes over many years. Long-term alcohol drinkers are also at high risk. Men are at higher risk than women, although this fact may simply reflect smoking and drinking habits in men. Over the past decade, multiple investigators have found a clear link between infection with certain strains of human papillomavirus (HPV) and development of cancer in the throat. When nonsmoking patients develop HNSCC, particularly in the oropharynx (upper throat/back of mouth), HPV should be suspected until proven otherwise. Patients with HPV-positive tumors have an improved overall survival relative to those with HPV-negative tumors. Since the HPV status is an independent predictor of outcome, HPV testing should be routinely performed on these tumors. The Epstein-Barr virus (EBV) has been linked to development of cancer of the nasopharynx.

Signs and Symptoms

The most common symptoms of HNSCC include persistent throat or ear pain, hoarseness, and/or significant voice changes. Patients may also present to their doctor with only a painless neck mass from an enlarged lymph node.

Diagnosis

Most patients will be seen initially by a primary care physician and referred to an ENT. This type of surgeon will generally perform a panendoscopy with the patient under sedation. This procedure involves placing a thin fiberoptic scope into the throat, in order to see the entire throat lining, including the larynx (voicebox). Biopsy may be performed during panendoscopy to confirm the presence or absence of cancer, as well as the type. For patients who have enlarged lymph nodes, biopsy may be performed under CT guidance. The vast majority of patients with head and neck cancer have squamous cell carcinoma. Less commonly, patients may have cancers that arise within the salivary glands and are called adenocarcinomas (the most common type of glandular cancer in the body; including breast, prostate, etc). Adenoid cystic cancers and other types are much less common.

Staging

Standard laboratory evaluation includes a complete blood count, serum chemistries, and may also include evaluation for blood levels of viruses including EBV in patients with suspected nasopharynx cancer. The levels of EBV in patients with advanced nasopharynx cancer should be monitored after completion of treatment since they can predict outcome. Patients who have persistently elevated EBV tend to have significantly worse survival than those who have no detectable blood levels after treatment. Most patients with HNSCC should undergo a CT of the neck and chest x-ray or chest CT to evaluate potential spread to the lungs or separate primary cancers originating from the lungs. Patients with HNSCC, particularly those who have been long-term smokers, are also at very high risk for both lung and esophageal cancers. MRI of the neck may be ordered to further evaluate the primary tumor. PET/CT is often ordered to evaluate potential spread to lymph nodes and/or distant, metastatic sites. A recent multicenter study revealed that PET improved the TNM staging and altered treatment recommendations in almost 15% of patients. PET can also be very helpful during RT planning.

There are several variations within the staging for each subsite of HNSCC (mouth, throat, voicebox, etc.) utilizing the AJCC TNM system. For further specifics, readers should refer to the *AJCC TNM Staging Manual, Seventh Edition.* However, there are common themes throughout the process. Patients whose cancers are small and confined to the site of origin have early stage disease. Those with large primary tumors that may invade other structures nearby and those that have spread to lymph nodes are considered to have locally advanced disease. Patients with metastatic HNSCC, most commonly to the lungs, liver, or bones, are generally incurable.

Treatment

Early stage cancers head and neck cancers are most commonly treated with surgery. A notable exception is early larynx cancer. These cancers are often treated with RT alone so that patients are able to keep their voicebox. The cure rates are about 90% with RT for early cancers of the vocal cords. Surgery carries risks of bleeding and infection, but most patients tend to do well following removal of small cancers in the head and neck region, particularly in the mouth or oral cavity. Recent surgical advances have decreased some side effects by using less invasive procedures. Long-term speech or swallowing problems are fortunately now less common. Side effects of RT for early larynx cancer include acute worsening of hoarseness and sore throat. Most patients will return to normal within a month or two after RT, though a very small percentage will have persistent hoarseness or chronic pain.

Not uncommonly, patients who undergo surgery for presumed early stage HNSCC are found to have more advanced disease following their surgery. This information is determined following review of the surgical specimen by a pathologist. The specimen usually includes the primary tumor as well as any lymph nodes that are removed from the neck. A subgroup of these patients will require postoperative RT and some will even require chemoRT. The latter group includes those patients who have multiple lymph nodes positive, extracapsular extension (cancer that extends beyond the capsule of the lymph node), and/or positive surgical margins (tumor cells extending to the edge of where the surgeon removed the cancer). Two major RCTs, one from the U.S. and one from Europe, revealed a survival benefit to chemoRT over RT alone for these groups of patients. Patients who require postoperative chemoRT are at high risk for tumor returning and dying of their cancer. Survival rates for HNSCC at five years after diagnosis range from 40% to 80%, varying by tumor (T) and nodal (N) stage.

Patients with locally advanced HNSCC, particularly those with primary tumors in the throat or larynx, are commonly treated without surgery for "organ preservation." Historically, organ preservation for patients with HNSCC was achieved with RT alone, though cure rates were not high. Therefore, radiation oncologists tested the use of a higher biologic dose of RT. Early RCTs revealed that RT using two fractions per day (to a higher total RT dose and/or over a shorter time course) was able to control cancer better than treatment with one RT fraction daily over seven weeks. Side effects were worse, but local tumor control was much better, and some patients had longer overall survival.

Another way that cancer specialists tested to improve cure rates was by adding chemotherapy to treatment regimens prior to RT, called "induction" chemotherapy. A famous study from the Department of Veterans Affairs revealed that patients treated with induction chemotherapy followed by RT had similar cure rates to laryngectomy (removal of the voicebox), but with the added benefit of keeping their larynx in about two-thirds of cases. Another RCT revealed a similar benefit to patients with advanced cancer of the pyriform sinus, an area within the hypopharynx next to the larynx. These studies dramatically changed the standard of care for patients, since most (all but the most advanced cancers) no longer required removal of their larynx for potential cure.

Other physicians and clinical researchers began testing RT alone versus RT plus chemotherapy at the same time, called concurrent chemoRT. Multiple RCTs and at least one meta-analysis (massive study evaluating the results of multiple RCTs together) have shown a significant benefit to chemoRT over RT alone in terms of local tumor control as well as survival. Concurrent chemoRT was then tested against induction chemotherapy followed by RT.

Concurrent treatment was proven superior in at least one RCT and one meta-analysis.

Thus, the current standard of care for most patients with locally advanced HNSCC is seven weeks of daily IMRT to a dose of about 70 Gy, delivered with concurrent cisplatin chemotherapy. The chemotherapy is commonly delivered in high doses once every three weeks. Lower doses of cisplatin delivered once per week work well also (often with less side effects in the author's experience). Cure rates are usually in the neighborhood of 70% to 80% long term. Among those patients who have their cancer return, the majority will do so in the first two to three years following completion of chemoRT. Development of distant metastases is a common scenario among patients who fail after chemoRT, either alone or in combination with local recurrence of tumor at the primary site (where the cancer started).

Acute side effects of RT to the head and neck region include skin reaction, sore mouth and/or throat, fatigue, and difficulty swallowing. Long-term potential side effects include dry mouth, swallowing problems, and a rare chance of focal injury to the jaw or other structures, requiring surgical repair. Over the past decade, widespread incorporation of IMRT for treatment of HNSCC has decreased the risk of permanent dry mouth (also called xerostomia), which was previously an almost guaranteed side effect of RT. Now radiation oncologists are usually able to minimize the RT dose that's delivered to one or both parotid glands, and spare more salivary function.

The most common chemotherapy used concurrently with IMRT is cisplatin. Acute side effects include fatigue, poor appetite, decreased blood counts, and nausea and vomiting, the latter of which is generally well controlled on current antibiotic of medicines. Less common but severe side effects after cisplatin chemotherapy include damage to kidneys or nerves, as well as loss of high-frequency hearing.

Patients who are unable to tolerate chemotherapy during RT may be offered a medicine called cetuximab concurrent with IMRT. Cetuximab is a type of targeted anti-cancer therapy called a monoclonal antibody (the "-mab" on the end of the word is the clue). It acts at an area on the surface of the cancer cell called the epidermal growth factor receptor (EGFR) and inhibits (blocks) this receptor to prevent tumor cell growth. At least two major RCTs have shown an overall survival benefit to the addition of concurrent cetuximab. The first trial tested RT with or without the drug, and the second trial tested chemoRT with or without cetuximab. The most prominent side effect of the drug is a rash that appears like a horrible case of teenage acne across the cheeks and face. Interestingly, patients who develop more severe rash also have a better outcome.

Patients with locally advanced HNSCC who receive chemoRT or RT with cetuximab as their definitive treatment sometimes have residual abnormalities remaining in their neck after treatment. It's not uncommon to have a residual small mass that can be either felt on physical examination or seen on imaging studies such as neck CT or PET/CT scans. The role of neck lymph node dissection (LND; removal of lymph nodes) in this situation is somewhat controversial. In years past, surgeons frequently planned LND to occur after chemoRT for any patients with large or multiple lymph nodes that were present at the beginning of treatment. Now, a frequent recommendation is for LND to be performed only for residual disease that can be felt on examination or seen on imaging studies two months after completion of treatment. Several reports indicate that the need for LND following chemoRT should be uncommon. It's important to give the chemoRT ample time to kill the tumors and for the body's immune system to remove dead cells from those areas.

In the past, the surgery that was most often performed for treatment of tumors in the neck in patients with HNSCC was called a modified radical neck dissection. This surgery had potential for significant side effects including long-term shoulder dysfunction, neck stiffness, and occasional severe injury to the main vein in the neck. Currently, selective LNDs are more limited, with rare shoulder problems or severe side effects. On the other hand, fibrosis and stiffness in the neck remains a problem for some patients. An RCT actually has shown a benefit for acupuncture in this setting to reduce pain and neck dysfunction.

Clarence's Head and Neck Cancer Treatment and Outcome

Clarence's ENT specialist sent him for a PET/CT scan, which confirmed abnormal activity in the tongue base and left neck but no other abnormal activity in the right neck or distantly.

Since his primary tumor was 4.5 cm, his single lymph node in the left neck was 2 cm, and he had no distant metastases evident, his final clinical stage was T3N1M0. His ENT referred him to a radiation oncologist and a medical oncologist, who recommended definitive chemoRT. Clarence underwent seven weeks of treatment which was very difficult. He received IMRT in order to minimize RT dose to his right parotid gland and any subsequent, long-term dry mouth. However, he did experience significant sore throat and some difficulty swallowing from the IMRT, which resolved about two months after the completion of treatment. His concurrent chemotherapy with cisplatin caused severe fatigue and some nausea, which was controlled with medicine. Examination during the final week of treatment revealed no palpable tumor remaining in the tongue base and minimal residual thickening in his left neck. Two months after chemoRT finished, he underwent a restaging PET/CT scan, which revealed no residual abnormal activity. Clarence has been seen by one of his cancer doctors every three months for the past three years and remains cancer free.

KIDNEY CANCER

Sally's Story

Sally was a 50-year-old personal trainer and former marathoner. The highlight of her day was her morning run. She was proud that her body fat percentage remained in the single digits. She had no significant past medical history and no family history of cancer. One day while running, she became acutely sick with nausea and severe abdominal pain. She went to the local emergency department, where examination revealed tenderness in her left lower abdomen. She was sent for a CT scan of the abdomen and pelvis which revealed inflammation in the colon. The doctor in the emergency department thought she might be suffering from an acute case of diverticulitis, an inflammation within pockets of tissue that can form in the colon. However, incidentally noted on the CT scan was a large mass occupying about 30% of her left kidney that clearly did not appear to be a cyst and was suspicious for cancer. She was admitted to the hospital, where her abdominal pain resolved over two days after lots of IV fluids and relative bowel rest. Sally was seen by a urologist, who agreed that the appearance of her left kidney on the CT scan was most consistent with a renal cell carcinoma, kidney cancer. Rather than a biopsy, her urologist recommended a radical nephrectomy, surgical removal of the kidney. (To be continued....)

Surprising to many people, kidney cancer is common. It's estimated that in 2010, 58,000 patients will be diagnosed and 13,000 will die of the disease in the United States. The median age at diagnosis is 64 years old, and it's rarely diagnosed before age 35. The lifetime risk of being diagnosed with cancer of the kidney is 1.5%, or about one in 70 people. According to the most recent NCI's SEER Cancer Statistics Review, the five-year survival, relative to the general population, following a diagnosis of kidney cancer for all stages combined is 69%. If the disease is localized, then the five-year survival for kidney cancer is 90%. Patients with regional spread to lymph nodes have a five-year survival rate of 63%. Those with distant, metastatic kidney cancer have an 11% survival rate at five years following diagnosis.

Risks and Causes

Most patients who develop cancer of the kidney have no known risk factors. Patients who are on dialysis to treat end-stage acquired renal cystic disease have an increased risk of kidney cancer. However, the absolute risk is low, at around 5%. A fairly uncommon disease, von Hippel-Lindau (VHL), carries a 70% lifetime risk of developing kidney cancer. On the bright side though, the discovery of the VHL gene has led to significant advances in the treatment of kidney cancer. Other risk factors for kidney cancer include tobacco smoking and exposure to certain chemicals and toxins.

Signs and Symptoms

Hematuria (painless blood in the urine) is the most common symptom of kidney cancer. Pain under the back low ribs (flank) or a palpable mass on physical examination occurs in about 50% of patients. The classic triad of all three of these symptoms (hematuria, flank pain, and a palpable flank mass) is much less common. Quite frequently, patients are found to have kidney cancer after CT imaging of the abdomen and pelvis that is obtained for other reasons (as in Sally's case above). In the 30% to 35% of patients who already have distant spread of their cancer at diagnosis, symptoms may be related to the site of metastasis in the lungs, bones, brain, or liver.

Diagnosis

Most patients who present with hematuria, persistent flank pain, or other worrisome symptoms are referred to a urologist, a surgeon specializing in care of patients with problems of the genitourinary (GU) tract. Following CT imaging, the diagnosis of kidney cancer may be highly suspected. These patients often go straight to nephrectomy (surgical removal of the kidney) by their urologist. Occasionally, patients undergo CT-guided biopsy of a kidney mass. Roughly 80% of kidney cancers are renal cell carcinomas (RCC). The most common subtype is clear cell, which makes up about 80% of RCCs. Papillary and chromophobe types are much less common but have a very good prognosis and low risk of metastasis. Occasionally other primary cancers, such as lung or breast, may metastasize (spread) to the kidneys.

Staging

Standard blood work should include complete blood count and serum chemistries. In addition, all patients with RCC should undergo a bone scan due to the high risk of metastasis to the bones. Early-stage cancer is confined to the kidney and has a survival ranging from 70% to 90%. Regional disease extends into the adjacent tissues, including major blood vessels and lymph nodes. Distant metastases occur most frequently in the lungs, bones, and brain, but renal cell cancer can spread to the liver or other sites. Survival five years after diagnosis with stage IV metastatic kidney cancer is approximately 10%.

Treatment

Standard surgical treatment for kidney cancer for many years has been radical nephrectomy. The procedure may be performed with open (standard) surgery, including a large incision over the flank, or may be performed laparoscopically. The latter technique may decrease the duration of hospital stay as well as postoperative pain significantly. In recent years, partial nephrectomy, removal of only a portion of the kidney, has become the standard surgery for most patients with kidney cancer. The other name for partial nephrectomy is "nephron-sparing surgery," since the kidney is made up of many nephrons or functional units. Over the past few years, laparoscopic partial nephrectomy has become the surgical treatment of choice for smaller kidney tumors (stage T1) at major urologic cancer centers. Tumor control and survival rates for these well-selected patients in experienced hands appear similar to prior experience with the open (nonlaparoscopic) partial nephrectomy procedure. The most common side effect immediately after surgery is acute renal failure (kidneys shutting down), which can occur in up to 10% of patients. Chronic renal insufficiency (kidneys not working well long-term) may also occur in a small percentage of patients as a late effect of surgery.

Treatment for locally advanced RCC consists of nephrectomy with consideration for postoperative systemic treatment. The same medicines are also used for patients with metastatic RCC (see below). There is no clear role for RT postoperatively, except in rare cases.

Metastatic kidney cancer is, unfortunately, fairly common. As opposed to many other cancer types, many patients with RCC that's already spread to distant sites actually live longer by having their primary tumor in the kidney(s) surgically removed. However, the mainstay of treatment for patients with metastatic RCC is systemic. For many years, immunotherapy was the standard treatment. Interleukin-2 (IL2) and interferon alpha (IFN) were the two most common drugs.

Over the past few years, however, a revolution has occurred in the systemic management of metastatic RCC. Improvements in the understanding of molecular pathways by which RCC acts in the human body have led to the development of several new classes of medicines. Three new classes of biologic agents are improving the survival and quality of life of patients with metastatic RCC. These medicines have been found to be quite effective when tested in RCTs against placebo, against immunotherapy with IFN, or in combination with IFN.

One class of these medicines is called tyrosine kinase inhibitors (TKIs), which are now used in the treatment of a few different types of cancer. The two most commonly used TKIs for kidney cancer are sorafenib and sunitinib. One large RCT revealed a survival benefit for sorafenib over placebo in patients who had progressive disease after prior treatment with IFN. Another RCT showed that sunitinib helped patients remain alive longer without a recurrence of their disease compared to IFN as first-line treatment. A newer TKI, pazopanib, was proven effective in a trial against placebo and was approved by the FDA last year. Common moderate side effects of the TKIs include fatigue, high blood pressure, diarrhea, and hand-foot syndrome, which each occur in about 10% of patients.

Another group of biologic agents that works by blocking a different cancer growth pathway is mTOR inhibitors. Examples are everolimus and temsirolimus. In a multicenter RCT involving over 600 patients, temsirolimus was proven to prolong patients' survival compared to IFN. However, the addition of temsirolimus in combination with IFN did not improve results. The other mTOR inhibitor, everolimus, improved patients' chances of surviving without disease recurrence in those who had already failed treatment with one of the TKIs. Fatigue, rash, mouth sores, and swelling of the legs are common side effects of the mTOR inhibitors.

Lastly, bevacizumab is a type of agent called a vascular endothelial growth factor (VEGF) inhibitor. This drug blocks abnormal blood vessel growth and normalizes the blood vessels around the tumor. Neovasculature (new blood vessels) formed by the tumor in order to sustain itself often shrinks away dramatically after treatment with bevacizumab. The drug has shown significant activity against RCC (as it has against several other types of cancer) when compared to placebo. However, when the combination of bevacizumab and IFN was compared with IFN alone in two RCTs, no significant survival benefit was proven. Common side effects include fatigue, poor appetite, high blood pressure, and protein in the urine.

Sally's Kidney Cancer Treatment and Outcome

After much consideration, Sally agreed to and underwent a left nephrectomy. Pathologic review revealed a 7 cm renal cell carcinoma, with negative surgical margins and no involvement of the adjacent tissues or blood vessels. No further treatment was recommended. She recovered uneventfully and returned to work as a personal trainer within three weeks. Sally remains cancer free five years postoperatively and has happily returned to her long distance running routine.

LEUKEMIA

Tim's Story

Tim was a 45-year-old banker who was in overall good health. In addition to his job, he enjoyed playing racquetball and spending time with his wife and two daughters. Over a period of about six weeks, he noticed that he wasn't able to keep up with his opponents on the racquetball court. He was winded after only 10-15 minutes of play, when previously he could play for an hour with no problem. He also seemed to be getting viral upper respiratory infections ("colds") that would hang on for months, which never happened to him in the past. Because of his progressive fatigue, he went to see his primary doctor, with whom he had a very good relationship. Although his physical examination showed only some mild tenderness of his sinuses and he appeared slightly pale, his bloodwork revealed a white blood cell count that was almost 10X the normal level. His doctor referred him to a medical oncologist, who performed further bloodwork as well as a bone marrow biopsy. Tests of his blood and bone marrow revealed evidence of acute myelogenous leukemia, AML. (To be continued....)

Leukemia is different than most of the other common cancers in this guide because it's a cancer of abnormal blood cells that arises in the bone marrow, the soft center of bones where new blood cells are formed. Since it affects the bone marrow and blood predominantly, leukemia is often referred to as a "liquid tumor." Most of the remaining common cancers in the guide are referred to as "solid tumors." An estimated 43,000 patients will be diagnosed with leukemia in the United States in 2010, and 22,000 patients will die of their disease. While the median age of diagnosis is 64, the disease strikes children as well as the elderly and may occur at any age in between. The lifetime risk of developing leukemia is 1.3%, or one in 78 people. According to the NCI's SEER Cancer statistics, the survival rate five years following diagnosis, relative to the general population, for all adult patients with leukemia is 54%. The cure rate for leukemia in adults is usually much lower than for children with the disease. In fact, the most common type of leukemia in children, called acute lymphocytic (ALL), has a cure rate of about 90%. The remainder of the discussion in this chapter focuses on leukemia in adults.

There are two main ways to classify leukemia: acute versus chronic, and myeloid versus lymphoid or lymphocytic. Chronic leukemias are a problem of too many mature abnormal blood cells, while acute leukemias are a problem of too many immature or early blood cells, sometimes called blasts. Myeloid (also called myelogenous or granulocytic) cells are very early blood cells that go on to become red blood cells, platelets, or a type of white blood cells called neutrophils during normal development. On the other hand, lymphoid or lymphocytic cells develop into different types of mature white blood cells called lymphocytes. So, the difference between myeloid and lymphoid leukemias is in the type of blood cell that's accumulating abnormally. Taking these two combinations of two choices together, there are four main types of adult leukemia: acute myeloid (AML), chronic myeloid (CML), acute lymphocytic (ALL), and chronic lymphocytic (CLL). The most common type of leukemia in adults is CLL, followed by AML, then CML and ALL. Although leukemias account for 30% of childhood cancers, they make up a much smaller percentage of the total number of adult cancer cases diagnosed each year.

Risks and Causes

Most patients who have a leukemia diagnosis don't have a known predominant risk factor in their medical history. Exposure to certain types of chemotherapy agents, the classic type being alkylating agents, can increase the risk of developing leukemia as early as two to five years after treatment. While many of these drugs are no longer used, drugs such as etoposide and cyclophosphamide (which are routinely used in the treatment of lung and breast cancers, respectively) still carry a risk of causing leukemia, albeit very small in absolute terms. Radiation, particularly if received at a young age, may significantly increase the risk of developing leukemia years later as well. There are certain chemicals which are known to be carcinogens (cancer-causing agents) that also dramatically increase the risk. In addition to the host of other cancers that it causes, smoking also increases the risk of leukemia. Patients with severe blood disorders and certain chromosomal or genetic abnormalities, notably Down syndrome, also have an increased risk.

Signs and Symptoms

Classic signs of acute leukemia include fatigue, bleeding, easy bruising, and recurrent infections. These problems are usually a result of too many leukemic cells in the bone marrow causing a relative lack of the different normal functional blood cells. However, most people who feel fatigued and/or are prone to recurrent infections don't have leukemia.

Diagnosis

Most frequently, patients present with one or more of the above symptoms to their primary physician, who orders a complete blood count, which is often (though not always) markedly abnormal. This finding will generally prompt a referral to a hematologist, a doctor who specializes in diseases of the blood. Most commonly in the United States, these doctors are also medical oncologists who are trained to treat most types of cancers. In addition to specialized blood tests, the hematologist/oncologist will usually perform a bone marrow biopsy. During this outpatient procedure, after numbing the area, the doctor places a needle into the back of the hip bone or pelvis (usually) to take a sample from deep inside the bone. This fragment of bone and aspirate of bone marrow liquid are then sent to a laboratory for pathologic analysis, which may include chromosomal testing. The pathologic review helps to determine the presence or absence of leukemia, as well as the subtype to guide treatment.

Staging

The traditional AJCC TNM System doesn't apply to leukemia staging. The French-American-British (FAB) and World Health Organization (WHO) classification schemes are two types of classification that have been used for AML in order to subtype the leukemia and help to guide treatment.

Leukemia Treatment and Outcome

CLL

According to the most recent NCI's SEER Cancer Statistics Review, the five-year survival rate following a diagnosis of CLL is 78%, the highest of the four main types of adult leukemias.

Historically, CLL was treated with a chemotherapy medication called chlorambucil. However, numerous single agents and multidrug combinations have been tried for treatment of patients with symptomatic CLL. Classes of medications that have resulted in reasonable responses include purine analogues, alkylating agents, and monoclonal antibodies. None of these treatments has shown a clear overall survival benefit for patients. In that regard, many patients who are diagnosed with CLL don't actually receive any treatment until/unless they develop symptoms. Often, if they're fortunate, they may remain without symptoms for years. Nevertheless, patients with advanced or progressive disease usually require treatment. The purine analogue fludarabine has been proven in several RCTs to be superior to multiagent chemotherapy. Fludarabine is generally well tolerated, with the main side effect being a decrease in blood counts. Lastly, a new medication called bendamustine has recently been shown to be quite effective against CLL. An RCT including over 300 patients tested chlorambucil versus bendamustine IV once per month for up to six cycles. Median survival without progression of CLL was almost 22 months for patients who received bendamustine versus 8 months for those treated with chlorambucil. Overall survival was not significantly different. Common side effects of bendamustine include fatigue, nausea, skin reaction, and decreased blood counts with risk for severe infection.

AML

This leukemia is actually a group of several subtypes. According to the most recent NCI's SEER Cancer Statistics Review, the five-year survival following a diagnosis of all types of AML combined is 24%, the lowest of the four main types of adult leukemias. The classic induction or initial chemotherapy regimen for patients with AML who are in good overall condition has been a combination of cytarabine and an anthracycline (daunorubicin, idarubicun, or mitoxantrone). A couple of studies have shown that idarubicin was the best of the anthracyclines in combination with cytarabine for induction. The chance of responding to induction chemotherapy is about 60% to 65%. Of this group, about 40% will go on to complete chemotherapy without a return of their disease. Therefore, about 25% of patients overall (0.60 x 0.40) will be alive and free of leukemia long term. Older patients tend to fare worse, as do those with a very high WBC, blood disorders, or leukemic cells in their nervous system. Cytogenetic or chromosomal studies on the blood and bone marrow samples also provide information that informs prognosis. Some of these chromosomal abnormalities are consistent with a better outcome, while some predict for a worse response to treatment and poor survival.

The treatment and outcome for younger patients with AML (generally less than 60 years old) has improved dramatically over the past decade. Patients who are fortunate to have a remission of leukemia following initial chemotherapy and are in good condition are generally offered aggressive treatment with high-dose chemotherapy. A couple of major RCTs revealed that after remission from induction chemotherapy, patients fared better with further high-dose cytarabine chemotherapy alone than with bone marrow transplantation afterward. Over the past few years, multiple other classes of systemic agents have proven to be effective against AML. These include inhibitors (blockers) of tyrosine kinase and farnesyl transferase.

CML

Systemic treatment for CML is one example of a modern medicine success story. This disease results classically (though not always) from a wrong movement of genetic pieces between chromosomes. The result of these two pieces, called BCR and ABL, moving together erroneously forms what is termed the Philadelphia chromosome, which is found to be present in many patients with CML. Historically, the disease was treated with a type of immunotherapy called interferon alpha (IFN) which didn't have great success and caused significant side effects for patients. However, over the past decade, thanks to advances in molecular biology, a new class of drugs has become the standard of care, resulting in better outcomes, including less toxicity from treatment. "Shotgun" treatment to the entire immune system with IFN has been replaced with targeted drug therapy using a class of tyrosine kinase inhibitors (TKIs). More specifically, a subgroup of TKIs that inhibits or blocks BCR-ABL has been shown to be much more effective than IFN in an RCT. The most common BCR-ABL inhibitor in use over the past several years has been imatinib. However, two major RCTs published just a couple of months ago revealed a significant benefit to second generation BCR-ABL inhibitors, nilotinib and dasatinib. These drugs have become the new standard for treatment of chronic phase CML that's Philadelphia chromosome positive. Other than decreases in blood counts, severe toxicities are rare with these medications. Common milder side effects of nilotinib and dasatinib include fatigue, headache, rash, fluid retention, and diarrhea. While CML still isn't cured in the majority of patients, these newer medications have increased patients' chances and decreased the side effects of treatment. According to the most recent NCI's SEER Cancer Statistics Review, the five-year survival following a diagnosis for CML is 57%.

ALL

As mentioned above, treatment of ALL in adults hasn't historically been as successful as treatment of childhood ALL. According to the most recent NCI's SEER Cancer Statistics Review, the five-year survival for adults with ALL is 65%. A multiagent chemotherapy regimen is used for treatment over a six- to nine-month initial course, followed by treatment of the central nervous system, because leukemia can relapse there commonly. Patients are then treated with a maintenance chemotherapy regimen over two years. Adult patients with ALL are considered to have high-risk disease and those who are in good condition should be considered for treatment with high-dose chemotherapy and bone marrow transplant. Until the past decade, results for adults with ALL were fairly disappointing. However, advances in supportive care have allowed more intensive treatment in adults. Five-year survival for adults with ALL is 40-50% in recent years. Moreover, for patients who are found to be Philadelphia chromosome positive, treatment directed at BCR-ABL with imatinib and the second generation TKIs is also improving outcomes.

Tim's Leukemia Treatment and Outcome

Tim received high-dose cytarabine and idarubicin induction chemotherapy. He was admitted to the hospital for treatment of febrile neutropenia, a condition where the white blood cells that fight infection are very low due to the high-dose chemotherapy. Tim received IV antibiotics and fluids, his fever resolved, and he made a full recovery. He was found to be in remission after induction chemotherapy, and then he received further high-dose cytarabine. Tim was in the fortunate group of patients whose disease never returned. Three years after completion of chemotherapy, he's back to enjoying a normal life with his wife and daughters. He's lost a step or two on the racquetball court but has absolutely no complaints.

LIVER CANCER

Joey's Story

Joey spent nearly his entire life on the road. After a very difficult childhood moving among various foster homes, he felt more comfortable on the move as an adult. Since the age of 25, he'd been a long-haul trucker. Although he enjoyed the money and the lifestyle, his body had begun to feel the pain of endless fast-food joints and bars. Joey was an alcoholic and had been hospitalized for bouts of pancreatitis in the past. He'd even tried rehab, but that didn't work. Now, at the age of 66, he felt like he was breaking down altogether. Over the past couple of years, he'd noticed that his belly was getting harder, and the spider-like veins that covered it seemed to show more every day. The past few months, Joey seemed even more tired than usual. It seemed like his belly was always full and he was rarely hungry. When he made a holiday stop to see an old lady friend, she was struck by how sick Joey looked. She convinced him to let her drive him to the hospital. The doctor at the emergency department noticed that Joey's skin appeared slightly jaundiced (yellow), his belly was hard, and he was able to feel his liver, which felt like a rock, extending well below his right ribcage. He agreed with Joey that the veins on his belly were prominent. The doctor ordered a CT scan of the abdomen, which revealed a small amount of ascites (abnormal fluid in the abdomen), as well as at least two masses in the liver. Joey underwent an MRI of the liver, which confirmed a

5 x 5 cm dominant mass in the right lobe just under the dome of the liver, as well as two other tumors that appeared to be 2-3 cm each in size. The left lobe of the liver appeared to be uninvolved. His alpha-fetoprotein (AFP) level in the blood was markedly elevated above the normal level. He was seen by a surgeon who specialized in hepatobiliary tumors (cancers of the liver and bile ducts). The surgeon told him that, based on his AFP level, he clearly had hepatocellular carcinoma, liver cancer. (To be continued....)

The situation with tumors involving the liver is similar to the brain. Metastases from other sites are much more common than primary liver tumors. Management of metastatic tumors to the liver is discussed in the chapter on colorectal cancer. In 2010 in the United States, primary cancers of the liver and bile ducts within the liver are estimated to be diagnosed in 24,000 patients. Within this group, about 75% arise from the liver tissue and these are predominantly hepatocellular carcinomas (HCC). Cancers of the bile ducts within and just outside the liver tissue, called cholangiocarcinomas, account for another 10% to 20%. It's estimated that 19,000 patients will die of these diseases each year in the United States. The median age at diagnosis is 64, and these diseases are rarely diagnosed before age 35. The lifetime risk of developing HCC is a 0.8%, or about one in 125 people.

According to the most recent NCI's SEER Cancer Statistics Review, the five-year survival following a diagnosis of liver cancer or bile duct cancer for all stages combined is 14%. If the disease is localized, then the five-year survival is 26%. Patients with regional spread to lymph nodes or distant, metastatic liver cancer have five-year survival rates of 9% and 3%, respectively. The discussion within the remainder of his chapter centers on HCC, since it's the most common primary liver cancer.

The five-year survival following a liver cancer diagnosis is 10% to 15% overall. Unfortunately, most HCCs develop in patients who've had cirrhosis (scarring of the liver tissue) for many years, if not decades. These patients are generally quite sick even before they develop cancer. They're not commonly able to tolerate major liver surgery and tend to fare quite poorly, accounting for the fairly dismal five-year survival rate noted above. About one third of patients present with disease that's localized. Patients who are in excellent condition and have small tumors usually are able to have surgery. This small group tends to have the best survival, approaching 50% at five years after diagnosis.

Risks and Causes

The most common risk factor for HCC is chronic hepatitis, inflammation of the liver leading to cirrhosis. After 20 to 30 years, the absolute risk of developing HCC is 1% to 3%. Chronic alcoholism is a common cause of cirrhosis, leading to HCC, but it's not the only cause. Chronic hepatitis B virus (HBV) increases the relative risk of developing HCC approximately 100 times over the general population, and it's the most common cause of HCC worldwide. However, in the United States, Hepatitis C virus (HCV) is the main risk factor for about 50% of patients who are diagnosed with primary liver cancer. While there's a vaccine for HBV, there isn't one for HCV, and there's no cure.

Although chronic HCV infection is common, the absolute risk of developing HCC is still quite small. Men are about three times more likely to be diagnosed than women. People living in parts of Africa and Southeast Asia are at much higher risk than in the United States, mainly due to chronic HBV infection and lack of vaccination. Obesity and diabetes are also risk factors for HCC. Lastly, athletes and others foolish enough to use anabolic steroids long-term significantly increase their risk of developing HCC compared to the general population. Therefore, for people fortunate enough to be born in countries like the United States, it's mainly lifestyle choices that affect the risk factors for development of HCC. These factors can clearly be modified.

Signs and Symptoms

The most common symptom for patients with liver cancer is abdominal pain. Jaundice (yellow skin) may also occur, particularly when cancers of the biliary tract cause mechanical blockage. Patients with more advanced disease may present to their doctor with complaints of weight loss and anorexia. Nausea and vomiting may also occur. Still others may be found to have ascites, fluid in the abdomen, caused by the cancer.

Diagnosis

In addition to a thorough physical examination, initial laboratory evaluation includes complete blood count, chemistries, liver function tests, and serum alpha-fetoprotein (AFP), as well as carcinoembryonic antigen (CEA) levels. Imaging may begin with an ultrasound, but usually includes CT of the abdomen with contrast. MRI of the liver delineates the anatomy quite well. PET/CT may be considered to evaluate for potential metastases. Diagnosis is often made based on imaging and an elevated AFP blood level. Biopsy may be performed by a surgeon, or by a radiologist using CT or ultrasound guidance.

Staging

The AJCC TNM system is used for liver cancer staging. The staging of HCC depends upon whether there are single or multiple lesions, as well as their size and location. Of particular importance is whether the tumor(s) invade or encase major blood vessels. In addition, the serum AFP and underlying severity of the patient's liver disease are important factors for their prognosis. As mentioned, those with severe cirrhosis tend to do relatively poorly.

Treatment

The main treatment for liver cancer (HCC) as well as cancers of the biliary tract is surgery. The tumor must be technically resectable, and the patient must be in good enough condition to undergo this major operation. Unfortunately, many patients aren't able to have surgery for one or both of these reasons. The two main categories of surgery for primary liver cancer are partial hepatectomy (removal of part of the liver) or orthotopic liver transplantation (OLT; liver transplant). GI specialists and surgeons classify patients who have cirrhosis according to a long-standing method called the Child-Pugh score or classification. Those with the best prospects for survival are class A, and the worst are class C. Another scoring system that's been used more recently by liver surgeons is the "model for end-stage liver disease," or MELD score. This system helps surgeons decide which patients are candidates for OLT, since a high MELD score predicts for a high chance of death after surgery. Pathologic factors that predict for worse survival include tumors that are large, high grade, multiple, or invading major blood vessels. Surgical risks include infection and significant bleeding. Liver surgery carries a higher mortality or death rate than most types of surgery. Patients who receive a liver transplant are placed on medicines that suppress the immune system, which puts them at high risk for life-threatening infection.

For patients who are unable or unwilling to undergo surgical resection, there are several other local treatment options. These include transarterial chemoembolization (TACE), radiofrequency ablation (RFA), and stereotactic body radiation therapy (SBRT). Transarterial chemoembolization involves delivery of anticancer drugs directly into the blood vessels of the liver. RFA involves the placement of probes or electrodes into the tumor and heating them with an electrical current in the range of radiowaves to kill cancer cells. Lastly, SBRT is a type of highly focused, high-dose RT delivered using CT and/or MRI planning and generally delivered over one to five days. Side effects of these treatments include a risk of infection, inflammation causing pain, flulike symptoms, and occasionally severe, life-threatening injury to the liver.

Most of the major RCTs for treatment of HCC come from Asia, since the incidence there is much higher than in the United States. An RCT from Taiwan comparing RFA versus ethanol injection revealed RFA to be superior for tumors 4 cm or less. Another trial randomized patients with resectable tumors to surgery with versus without preoperative TACE. This trial failed to show a significant improvement for the patients that received the preoperative TACE. Lastly, a large RCT from China compared TACE alone versus RFA alone versus the TACE-RFA combination for the treatment of tumors larger than 3 cm. This trial revealed that the median survival for patients treated with the TACE-RFA combination was 37 months, as opposed to 24 and 22 months for TACE and RFA, respectively. Therefore, the standard of care for patients with large HCCs in China is now the combination of TACE and RFA. This combination is used for many patients in the United States and elsewhere who are poor candidates for surgery.

Systemic treatment for HCC is limited in its effectiveness. Standard chemotherapy doesn't work well. Newer biologic agents have shown some effectiveness. These include erlotinib and sorafenib, both of which are in a class of drugs called kinase inhibitors. These medicines are generally offered to patients who have poor liver function and extensive cancer, usually after local options are exhausted.

Joey's Liver Cancer Treatment and Outcome

After examining Joey and reviewing his scans and bloodwork, the surgeon told him that he felt surgery would be too risky for him. He told Joey that his cirrhosis from chronic alcohol abuse was too severe. The surgeon explained that some patients can tolerate the removal of the entire right side of their liver, but their remaining liver needs to be in good shape which Joey's wasn't. Joey's family asked about a liver transplant, but the surgeon explained that's a good option for people who have less cancer in their liver, if they're able to avoid drinking alcohol for six months to let their liver get in better condition. Joey told him bluntly that wasn't going to happen in any case. His GI specialist recommended TACE in combination with RFA, to which Joey agreed. He received two TACE treatments, which he tolerated well and which resulted in improvement of his liver function. RFA was able to shrink down two of the lesions. Joey continued binge drinking heavily over the following months, and his cirrhosis worsened. A repeat MRI scan of the liver one year after initial treatment revealed multiple small new tumors in the liver. The medical team offered systemic treatment with a medicine called sorafenib. However, Joey decided against further treatment. He died 18 months after his initial diagnosis.

LUNG CANCER

Billy's Story

Billy was a 71-year-old commercial fisherman who lived life hard. He smoked two packs of cigarettes each day and drank a fifth of whiskey every two days. However, he was strong and motivated enough that he continued to work full time. He developed a cough that wouldn't go away. In addition, he'd been getting terrible headaches each morning that made it tough to get through his routine on the boat. He finally decided he'd better go to the local medical clinic. His examination revealed high blood pressure and a crackling sound in the bottom of his right lung. Due to Billy's worrisome symptoms and his being a nearly life-long smoker, the doctor on duty recommended a chest x-ray and CT scan of his head. The chest x-ray revealed a mass in the central right lung. CT of the brain revealed an abnormality in the back of the left part of the brain. CT of the chest confirmed a 3 cm mass in the right lung with two smaller masses in the left lung, each measuring less than 1 cm, all worrisome for cancer. The remainder of the brain was unremarkable. Billy was referred to a pulmonologist (lung specialist). He performed a bronchoscopy, a procedure that involves passing a thin fiberoptic scope down the trachea (windpipe) in order to see the bronchial tree (major airways) in the central lungs. The lung doctor saw a mass pushing on the outside of the right main bronchus. Biopsy during the bronchoscopy revealed an adenocarcinoma, nonsmall-cell cancer of the lung. (To be continued....)

Thanks mainly to the widespread use of tobacco products, and cigarettes in particular, lung cancer is extremely common. It's the leading cancer killer in the world. It's estimated that 223,000 patients will be diagnosed and 157,000 will die of lung cancer in 2010 in the United States. While the median age at diagnosis is around 70 years old, lung cancer occurs in patients in their 40s and 50s regularly, particularly those who start smoking in their teenage years. The lifetime risk of developing lung cancer is 7%, or one in 14 people. Of course, these risks differ dramatically, depending upon whether a person is regularly exposed to tobacco smoke or not.

According to the NCI's SEER Cancer Statistics Review, the five-year survival rate for lung cancer for all stages combined is a rather dismal 16%. Only about 15% of patients have localized disease when they are diagnosed. Their chance of survival at five years following a lung cancer diagnosis is 53%, relative to the general population. Those with locally advanced disease have a five-year survival of 24%. Patients who have metastatic lung cancer that's already spread to distant sites at the time of diagnosis have a 4% chance of surviving five years. Clearly there's ample room for improvement in the fight against lung cancer.

Risks and Causes

Approximately 90% of patients who are diagnosed with lung cancer have a history of smoking. The rest develop lung cancer as a result of exposure to secondhand smoke or other known carcinogens including radon. Other studies have recently shown an increased risk of lung cancer diagnosis and/or death for women using long-term hormone replacement therapy with estrogen and progesterone. Chronic inflammation as measured by blood levels of C-reactive protein also appears to double the risk of a lung cancer diagnosis.

Signs and Symptoms

Many symptoms of lung cancer unfortunately are similar to those of upper respiratory infections, including bronchitis or pneumonia. These include cough, dyspnea (shortness of breath), chest pain, and occasionally blood-tinged sputum. Many patients with these symptoms are initially treated with a course of antibiotics for presumed bronchitis. Others who have a history of chronic obstructive pulmonary disease (COPD) may be treated with bronchodilators and/or steroids ("inhalers") by their primary doctor or pulmonologist. The vast majority of patients will have their symptoms resolve after these medications, since most of the time the source will be infection or lung inflammation. However, symptoms that don't resolve always require further investigation. Unexplained weight loss, a cough that persists for more than a couple of weeks, or hemoptysis (coughing up blood) should always prompt medical attention. Still other patients are found to have lesions on chest x-rays or CTs of the chest obtained for other purposes and are asymptomatic (without symptoms) at the time. This group of patients tends to fare better than those who already have symptoms.

Diagnosis

It's extremely common for patients to have a chest x-ray that reveals a mass and prompts further evaluation with a CT of the chest. If the CT scan confirms a lung mass suspicious for cancer, then a CT-guided biopsy may be performed by a radiologist for diagnosis. PET/CT scans may also be performed to further evaluate suspicious lung lesions that are seen on CT, prior to biopsy. Some masses are so suspicious that direct surgical resection is recommended. Lung cancer diagnosis can also be made by bronchoscopy (as noted in Billy's story above). If the tumor is visualized within the bronchial tree, then it may be biopsied. More recently, a procedure called endoscopic bronchial ultrasound (EBUS) has been shown to be fairly accurate with diagnosis by biopsying not only primary lung lesions but also enlarged lymph nodes in the mediastinum, the area in the center of the chest between the lungs. Approximately 75% of lung cancers are nonsmall cell (NSCLC). Most of the remaining 25% are small cell lung cancers. This differentiation is important since treatment of the two different types may be quite different.

Staging

The standard laboratory tests include complete blood counts, serum chemistries including kidney and liver function tests. After pathologic diagnosis has been determined, lung cancer staging consists of imaging with CT of the abdomen and a bone scan or PET/CT in order to evaluate potential spread in the body. MRI is the standard test for evaluating potential brain metastases, which are fairly common with lung cancer. The AJCC TNM staging system is utilized. For lung cancer staging, the system is based not only on tumor size but also on location of the primary tumor, the different lymph node sites within the chest, and the presence or absence of distant metastases. Unfortunately, about 75% of patients have either stage III or IV disease at the time of diagnosis. According to the AJCC, the five-year survival following diagnosis is 70% for stage I, 40% for stage II, 20% for stage III, and 1% to 3% for stage IV, metastatic lung cancer.

Occasionally, a procedure called a mediastinoscopy may be performed by a thoracic surgeon during lung cancer diagnosis or staging. During this procedure, the surgeon makes a small incision in the notch above the collarbone, and inserts a rigid scope. The surgeon is able to see and possibly biopsy multiple groups of lymph nodes in the center of the chest, where lung cancer often spreads. The procedure is most frequently performed to ensure no extensive involvement of these lymph nodes prior to any planned lung surgery.

In addition to staging, prognostic factors for lung cancer that may predict a patient's survival include the patient's overall condition, age, sex (male is worse), and PET scan intensity. There are also multiple biologic factors that may indicate how well the tumor will respond to treatment.

Treatment

NSCLC

Patients with early stage NSCLC who are medically fit for surgery should have it, usually in the form of a lobectomy. In this procedure, the thoracic surgeon removes the entire lobe of either lung that contains the primary tumor. There are three lobes in the right lung and two main lobes in the left. Previous trials have tested whether it suffices to perform a wedge resection, removal of only the tumor with a small margin of normal tissue around it (like a lumpectomy in the treatment of breast cancer). However, that type of surgery has resulted in a high risk of lung cancer returning when compared to standard lobectomy. Occasionally pneumonectomy, resection of the entire lung, is recommended due to the size or central location of a lung cancer. Patients who are in otherwise excellent shape and have good lung function may tolerate this procedure and be cured. Prior to lobectomy or pneumonectomy, thoracic surgeons will evaluate patients' heart and lung function thoroughly. In addition to obtaining objective lung function tests, some surgeons have been known to walk up and down stairs with patients to check their endurance. The major acute risks of this type of lung cancer surgery include bleeding and infection, as well as a small risk of respiratory failure of the remaining lung resulting in death.

There have been multiple RCTs testing the role of chemotherapy after lung cancer surgery for patients with stage I-III NSCLC. Most of the RCTs as well as a meta-analysis (that included over 8,000 individual patients from 34 trials) have shown a survival benefit to the addition of postoperative chemotherapy. It's now recommended to all but the earliest stage I patients or those in very poor condition. On the other hand, the role of postoperative RT is much more controversial. Common indications for RT after lobectomy include positive surgical margins or cancer involving the lymph nodes in the mediastinum in the center of the chest. When good radiation techniques are used, there does appear to be a benefit of RT after surgery even for some patients with earlier stage disease.

Some patients who have early stage lung cancer are unable to undergo surgery due to their poor overall condition or poor lung function, usually as a result of many years of heavy smoking. They are said to be medically inoperable. For these patients, stereotactic body radiation therapy (SBRT) can be an excellent form of treatment that results in over 90% tumor control. SBRT delivers a very high radiation dose to a focal area, usually over one to five treatment days. Severe side effects are very uncommon. Radiofrequency ablation (RFA) is another local type of treatment that may be recommended for these patients.

As mentioned earlier, approximately 75% of patients with NSCLC are diagnosed with either stage III or incurable stage IV disease. Several decades ago, RT alone to moderate doses was the standard recommendation for patients with stage III disease. Local tumor control was fair and long-term survival was rare. Therefore, in an attempt to improve cure rates, doctors and researchers tested giving chemotherapy prior to RT, so called "induction" chemotherapy. A significant survival benefit was seen over RT alone. However, subsequent RCTs revealed a survival benefit to concurrent chemoRT over sequential chemotherapy followed by RT. The current standard of care for most patients with stage III NSCLC is concurrent chemoRT. RT is delivered in daily fractions, five days per week, over six-and-a-half to seven weeks, to a dose of 60-75 Gy. Perhaps the most studied chemotherapy doublet in the setting of concurrent RT to the chest is cisplatin and etoposide. This combination is effective against both NSCLC and small cell types of lung cancer. Another common combination is carboplatin and paclitaxel.

Acute side effects of RT to the lung include skin reaction, fatigue, and sore throat that may cause difficulty swallowing solid foods. Esophagitis (inflammation of the esophagus) is a common toxicity of chest RT, since the esophagus is often next to cancerous lymph nodes that must be included within the high-dose RT region. A classic but less common side effect of RT to the lung is called pneumonitis. It's characterized by the patient developing a dry cough, low grade fever, and shortness of breath that usually occurs from one to three months after the course of RT is completed. In most patients, a course of oral steroid medication resolves the symptoms over a few weeks. Occasionally, a longer course of steroids is required for complete resolution. Long-term, there is a very low risk of permanently worsened breathing, including oxygen dependency, due to fibrosis or scarring of the lung. Severe damage to nerves or other tissues is rare.

Patients with metastatic lung cancer who are in otherwise reasonable condition often benefit from systemic chemotherapy. Much to the surprise of many patients and family members alike, chemotherapy for lung cancer actually has been proven in multiple trials to improve rather than hurt patients' quality of life. Most patients are treated with two different chemotherapy medicines at the same time, a so-called doublet, and usually tolerate the treatment very well. There are many different effective regimens. The combinations of cisplatin and etoposide as well as carboplatin and paclitaxel are used frequently (as they are for patients with stage III disease). Chemotherapy specialists usually recommended treatment with these two-drug regimens for patients who are in good overall condition. Those who are in worse condition may be treated with a single drug, rather than two at once. Other chemotherapy agents active in the treatment of NSCLC include gemcitabine, vinorelbine, docetaxel, and irinotecan. The duration of chemotherapy for patients with advanced or metastatic NSCLC is variable. Many medical oncologists recommend an initial two to four cycles, followed by restaging CT or PET/CT scans to evaluate how well the cancer is responding to treatment.

Over the past decade, a few targeted therapies have proven beneficial for the treatment of lung cancer. This group of medications is not chemotherapy, but it is systemic anticancer treatment. One good example of a successful targeted therapy is bevacizumab, an agent that attaches to the vascular endothelial growth factor (VEGF) receptor on cancer cells. This drug acts by normalizing the blood vessels around the tumor. Specifically, neovasculature (new blood vessels) formed by the tumor in order to keep itself alive may shrink away dramatically after treatment with bevacizumab. It's shown reasonable activity against NSCLC. In fact, an RCT revealed a survival benefit when bevacizumab was added to carboplatin and paclitaxel chemotherapy for patients with stage IIIb, IV, or recurrent NSCLC.

Another recent major RCT revealed a survival benefit to patients with lung cancer from a different type of targeted therapy called gefitinib. This medicine is an epidermal growth factor receptor (EGFR) blocker, a subtype of tyrosine kinase inhibitor (TKI). Some patients with NSCLC will have EGFR mutations on their tumors. Therefore, they would potentially benefit from medications to block EGFR receptors, in order to stop growth of these tumor cells. Therefore, doctors tested gefitinib versus standard chemotherapy with carboplatin and paclitaxel in a group of more than 200 such patients with metastatic lung cancer. The group who received gefitinib had a doubling of their survival without tumor returning compared to the group who received chemotherapy. EGFR inhibitors also have proven efficacy in the treatment of patients with recurrent NSCLC (lung cancer that's returned despite chemotherapy). Common side effects include rash that looks like bad acne, poor appetite, and elevation of liver blood tests.

Small Cell Lung Cancer

As opposed to patients with early stage NSCLC, those who have early or limited stage small cell lung cancer don't require surgery. Because small cell lung cancer is usually extremely responsive to chemotherapy and RT, concurrent chemoRT is the treatment of choice. The most widely used and successful chemotherapy regimen is cisplatin and etoposide. Thoracic RT is most effective when started during the first or second cycle of chemotherapy. A major RCT revealed that RT delivered twice per day in smaller doses over three weeks to a total dose of 45 Gy improved patients' survival versus treatment once per day to the same dose over five weeks. Since small cell cancer cells divide more rapidly than other cancers, it's not surprising that treatment with both chemotherapy and twice-daily RT is more effective than a less aggressive course.

Acute side effects of this chemotherapy include fatigue, poor appetite, decreased blood counts, and nausea and vomiting, the latter of which is generally well controlled on medicines. Less common but severe side effects include damage to kidneys or nerves as well as loss of high frequency hearing. Side effects of lung RT are as mentioned for NSCLC.

Since small-cell lung cancer has an extremely high risk of spread to the brain, RT is often used in low doses to the brain in order to decrease the risk of spread there. Two major RCTs have been completed in which half of the patients were randomized to receive prophylactic cranial irradiation (PCI) while the other half were not. The first trial included patients who received chemoRT for limited stage disease and had an excellent response. The second RCT included patients with extensive-stage small-cell lung cancer (that had spread to other sites) who had an excellent response to initial chemotherapy. Both trials revealed not only a decrease in the risk of cancer developing in the brain, but also an overall survival benefit to those patients who received PCI. This standard treatment to the whole brain is delivered over two weeks to a low dose of 25 Gy. The most common short-term side effects of PCI include alopecia (hair loss), scalp irritation, and mild fatigue, all of which are usually temporary. The most common long-term risk is problems with short-term memory or complex thinking which may vary significantly by the patient. There's also clear evidence that chemotherapy may cause poor long-term brain function including short-term memory loss. Some patients refer to this effect as "chemo brain."

Billy's Lung Cancer Treatment and Outcome

Following Billy's bronchoscopy, which confirmed NSCLC, he underwent a PET/CT, which revealed abnormal activity in the right middle lobe mass, two other nodules in the left lung that were less than 1 cm in size, three abnormal lymph nodes

---

in the center of the chest, and a questionable 1 cm lesion in the liver. The PET/CT scan did not evaluate his brain. (For discussion of the management of Billy's brain metastasis, please refer to "Billy's Story" in the chapter on brain metastases.) He was referred to a medical oncologist who recommended systemic treatment with carboplatin and paclitaxel chemotherapy. Billy reluctantly accepted the recommendation at the urging of his wife and daughter. He was surprised that after four cycles of chemotherapy, he actually felt much better than when he was initially diagnosed. Because he had heard many horror stories about people getting terribly ill with chemotherapy, he was expecting much worse. He did have some mild aching of his joints during the treatments as well as temporary decreases in his blood counts that made him feel weak for a few days each month. Billy did well for almost a year, at which time he underwent a repeat CT scan of the chest and abdomen. This study revealed multiple new nodules in both lungs as well as three lesions in the liver, all of which were consistent with a recurrence of his cancer. Restaging brain MRI revealed no new lesions there. His medical oncologist recommended a second-line chemotherapy regimen which kept his cancer from progressing for another six months, at which time the nodules in the lungs began to grow rapidly. Billy was feeling quite fatigued by this point, physically, mentally, and emotionally. He and his family decided upon supportive care with help from the community hospice. Billy died at home with his daughter at his bedside one month later.

LYMPHOMA—NON-HODGKIN

Mary's Story

Mary was a 69-year-old retired seamstress who loved to garden and spend time with her many children and grandchildren. She had a history of diabetes, which was controlled with oral medication, but was otherwise in reasonable health. When Mary's husband was giving her a kiss on the cheek, he felt a lump in the right side of her neck, just below the angle of her jaw. It was about the size of a grape, somewhat rubbery, and not at all painful. They were both concerned, so they made a trip to their family doctor. She felt the lump and treated her with a two-week course of antibiotics, figuring that the lymph node may be enlarged due to infection. However, it did not respond to the medication. Mary was sent to a general surgeon, who removed the entire lymph node during an outpatient surgical biopsy. After pathologic review, it was determined to contain diffuse large B cells consistent with an aggressive non-Hodgkin lymphoma. (To be continued....)

Non-Hodgkin lymphoma (NHL) is a much more common cancer than most people realize. It's not just one disease, but more like a group of diseases. NHL will be diagnosed in 66,000 patients and 20,000 patients will die in the United States in 2010. The lifetime risk of an NHL diagnosis is about 2%, or one in 50 people. According to the most recent NCI's SEER Cancer Statistics Review, the five-year survival following a diagnosis of NHL is 67%, relative to the general population. If the disease is localized, then the five-year survival is 81%. Patients with regional spread have a five-year survival rate of 71%. Those with stage IV lymphoma have a 58% survival rate at five years following diagnosis.

Risks and Causes

The most common risk factor for development of NHL is a poor or compromised immune system. Certain chemicals may also place patients at increased risk.

One specific type of NHL which is usually not aggressive, is highly curable, and occurs most often in the stomach is called mucosa associated lymphoid tissue (MALT). It results from an infection by an organism known as *Helicobacter pylori*. The discovery of this association between a bacterial infection and the development of gastric MALT lymphoma led to a medical treatment regimen which has relatively few side effects and cures the vast majority of patients. It's a success story of modern medical diagnosis and treatment!

Signs & Symptoms

Lymphoma may present in many ways. One of the most common presentations is painless enlargement of one or more lymph nodes. Many groups of lymph nodes exist throughout the body. Among those sites that patients may see or feel, there are large numbers of lymph nodes in the neck, under the arm, and in the groin. Many other lymph nodes exist deeper within the chest, abdomen, and pelvis, where they can't be seen or felt. The normal role of the lymph nodes is predominantly to capture potentially dangerous or infectious cells, limit their spread, and allow the body's immune cells to combat the invaders. The vast majority of patients who develop enlarged lymph nodes have an infection or inflammation as the source rather than lymphoma or another type of cancer. Nevertheless, enlarged lymph nodes that persist for more than a couple of weeks should prompt a visit to a doctor for further evaluation.

Other classic symptoms of lymphoma are called "B symptoms" and include fever higher than 101 degrees Fahrenheit, weight loss of more than 10% of body weight, and/or drenching night sweats. The presence of these symptoms should be recorded by the patient's doctors, since they're generally an indicator of more advanced systemic disease.

Diagnosis

Lymph nodes or other sites in the body suspected of containing lymphoma should ideally be surgically removed by excisional biopsy (complete removal of the whole lymph node or mass) whenever safe and feasible. Removing a sizeable amount of the abnormal tissue will provide the pathologist the most information to review, in order to best determine the presence or absence of lymphoma, as well as the subtype of lymphoma, which will guide treatment. As opposed to many other kinds of cancer, lymphoma has multiple subtypes. The two main types are Hodgkin and NHL. Hodgkin lymphomas are much less common (and aren't included in this guide for that reason) but the vast majority of patients are cured with chemotherapy and RT. The simplest way to classify NHL is into two groups: indolent (slow-growing), the majority of which are follicular cell types, versus aggressive, the majority of which are diffuse large B cell types. In addition to the type of lymphoma, the grade is important. Grade is a measure of the level of aggressiveness of the tumor cells and their degree of difference from normal cells. Grade 1 tumors are cancerous but only slightly different than normal cells. Grade 3 tumors are the most different from normal cells and potentially the most aggressive, fastest-growing types of cancers. Grade 2 tumors are intermediate in their level of aggression and growth rate. There are too many specific types of NHL to list here. Suffice it to say, however, that the correct pathologic diagnosis is critical. Treatment regimens and cure rates may differ significantly.

Staging

Laboratory testing should consist of complete blood count, serum chemistries including kidney and liver function tests, lactate dehydrogenase (LDH), as well as consideration for HIV testing in patients who have risk factors for infection. Imaging generally includes CT of chest, abdomen, and pelvis. After diagnosis of an aggressive type of NHL, PET/CT is recommended for further lymphoma staging. Biopsy of bone marrow should also be performed for all patients with follicular lymphoma due to the high risk of microscopic cancer cells being present at the time of diagnosis. Patients with advanced stage, aggressive lymphomas also generally undergo bone marrow biopsies.

The Ann Arbor System is used for lymphoma staging. Although it differs from the standard TNM system that is utilized for most cancers, the Ann Arbor system is detailed in the AJCC Cancer Staging Manual. It's based on the number and location of sites involved with lymphoma as well as the presence or absence of B symptoms, which are described above. In addition to the classic Ann Arbor Staging, prognostic indices have been developed for patients with lymphoma that help to predict survival. For patients with diffuse or aggressive NHL, the International Prognostic Index (IPI) score is used. The IPI is a five-point scale that is based on age, stage, LDH, the number of extranodal sites (areas of the body involved with disease outside of lymph nodes), and patient performance status or overall condition. For patients with follicular NHL, the follicular lymphoma international prognostic index (FLIPI) is based on age, stage, LDH, number of extranodal sites, and serum hemoglobin (an indicator of the presence or absence of anemia included in the complete blood count). In general, the more of these factors that are present, the higher the risk of dying of lymphoma. For instance, a patient with aggressive diffuse large B cell lymphoma who is more than 60 years old with stage IV disease, an elevated LDH blood level, and three sites of extranodal disease will tend to fare more poorly than a younger patient with early stage disease who has a normal serum LDH and no extranodal lymphoma present on physical examination or imaging studies.

Treatment

Aggressive lymphomas, such as the common diffuse large B cell type, are treated with combination chemotherapy, with or without radiation therapy (RT). The combination chemotherapy consists of cyclophosphamide, doxorubicin (H-daunorubicin), vincristine (Oncovin), and prednisone. The acronym for this combination is CHOP. Many RCTs over the past several decades have tested CHOP against multiple other multidrug chemotherapy regimens. None has proven superior and CHOP remains the standard. For patients whose lymphoma cells contain the receptor called CD-20, a medication called rituximab is prescribed. Rituximab is a type of anti-cancer treatment called a monoclonal antibody (the clue is the ending of the word in "-mab"), a subtype of targeted therapy. These specialized medicines aren't chemotherapy, but they're an excellent form of treatment for lymphomas. They attach to cancer cells and prevent them from growing or multiplying. Rituximab has few major side effects, although it's quite expensive. When rituximab is added to CHOP chemotherapy, the acronym for this regimen is called R-CHOP. It's the most commonly prescribed systemic therapy for patients with aggressive NHL in the United States. Depending upon the initial lymphoma stage and the response to chemotherapy, most patients receive between three and eight cycles of R-CHOP. Acute side effects may include fatigue, decreased blood counts, nausea and vomiting (usually well controlled with current anti-nausea medicines), body aches, and sometimes numbness of the hands or feet. Allergic reactions may occur but are uncommon. Rare but serious side effects following R-CHOP include severe worsening of heart function, long-term nerve injury, as well an increased risk of developing a cancer due to treatment years later.

Most patients with early stage, aggressive lymphomas should receive low-dose, involved field radiation therapy (IFRT) after completion of chemotherapy. IFRT is delivered in low doses because lymphoma cells are generally very responsive to RT. IFRT is usually directed at the sites of initial lymphoma involvement and immediately adjacent areas. The entire course of RT may be completed in three or four weeks, rather than the six- or seven-week course required for treatment of many other cancers. Trials have suggested an improvement in survival without a return of lymphoma for patients treated with the combination of CHOP chemotherapy followed by IFRT versus those treated with chemotherapy alone.

Side effects depend upon where the RT beams are aimed (usually the sites of initial disease) but include skin irritation and fatigue. Sore throat and difficulty swallowing may occur acutely when lymph nodes in the neck or mediastinum (center of the chest) are treated. When the treatment area is in or near the lungs, there's a low risk of radiation pneumonitis, which is a lung inflammation that classically occurs one to three months after treatment. It's characterized by low-grade fever, shortness of breath, and dry cough. The symptoms usually resolve following a course of steroids over a few weeks. A rare subset of patients may develop a secondary cancer years after RT. Those most at risk for radiation-induced cancers are patients treated at a younger age. For instance, teenage girls treated to the chest have a significantly increased risk of breast cancer developing 10 to 20 years after treatment. Patients who smoke cigarettes and receive RT to the chest have an even higher long-term risk of developing lung cancer than those who smoke but haven't received RT.

Patients who have advanced stage, diffuse large B cell cancer or other aggressive lymphoma types usually receive R-CHOP. Whether RT is recommended is dependent upon the response of tumor to the systemic therapy. Oncologists will generally prescribe several doses or cycles of chemotherapy, and then reevaluate the response of the lymphoma to the treatment with a PET/CT scan. Cure rates range from more than 80% for early stage disease in favorable patients, down to less than 40% for patients with more advanced disease in worse condition.

If patients have their disease return despite aggressive treatment, sometimes they can still be cured with further high dose chemotherapy followed by bone marrow transplantation. This highly specialized, aggressive type of treatment eliminates the patient's existing cancerous bone marrow and replaces it with new marrow that contains no cancer cells. This clean bone marrow is often taken from a person who is free of cancer but has very similar blood to the patient with lymphoma, such as a brother or sister.

Patients who are diagnosed with indolent, follicular lymphoma are often in a unique situation among patients with cancer. Frequently patients have stage III or IV disease at diagnosis. The chemotherapy agents that are used for late stage, follicular lymphoma may improve quality of life for those who have symptoms, but patients' overall lifespan may not be affected by the treatment. The most commonly utilized single agent in this setting is fludarabine. The combination of cyclophosphamide, vincristine, and prednisone (CVP) is the most common multi-drug regimen. Even though patients with stage III and IV follicular lymphoma may not be curable, they may live with their disease for many years. That's fairly rare with other cancers.

Patients who have early stage follicular lymphoma may be treated with low-dose IFRT with a small risk of side effects. The treatment is generally delivered over three to four weeks, to a dose of 30-36 Gy. This group of patients has a median survival from the time of diagnosis of almost 15 years in some reports, although many will have their lymphoma return in other sites of the body. The exception to this treatment guideline is patients with high-grade follicular large-cell lymphomas. They should generally be treated similar to patients with aggressive diffuse large cell lymphomas, with combination chemotherapy followed by IFRT for the best chance of cure.

Mary's Lymphoma Treatment and Outcome

After her biopsy, Mary underwent a PET/CT scan, which revealed abnormal activity in the right neck in multiple lymph nodes, but no other abnormal activity in the remainder of her body. She was seen by a medical oncologist, who performed a bone marrow biopsy that revealed no cancer cells. This specialist recommended R-CHOP chemotherapy. He referred her for radiation oncology consultation, where the doctor recommended RT after completion of her chemotherapy. Since she had no B symptoms and her abnormal lymph nodes were in two different areas in the right neck, her Ann Arbor stage was IIA. She tolerated the R-CHOP fairly well, but had expected fatigue and a decrease in her blood count that required a transfusion after her second treatment. A restaging PET/CT scan revealed only faint residual activity in one lymph node in her right neck. She received low dose IFRT over three-and-a-half weeks to the region which she tolerated with only a mild sore throat that resolved two weeks after finishing treatment. Mary has been followed closely by both her medical and radiation oncologists for four years with no evidence of lymphoma.

MELANOMA

Dale's Story

Dale was a 39-year-old graphic artist. He worked for a major marketing company but also did artwork for custom cars and choppers on the side. He had no significant past medical history except for multiple sunburns as a child. He grew up in Florida, where his parents both encouraged him to be outside, though he failed to use sunscreen regularly. Dale's girlfriend noticed a dark-colored patch on the top of his back, just behind his right shoulder. She was concerned and made him an appointment with a dermatologist. On examination, the doctor found a 3 x 1 cm blue-black lesion that was slightly raised above the skin surface. She performed a skin biopsy in her office which revealed melanoma. (To be continued….)

While not nearly as common as nonmelanoma skin cancer, melanoma is the most common deadly skin cancer. In 2010 in the United States, it's estimated that 68,000 patients will be diagnosed and 9,000 patients will die of their disease. The median age at diagnosis is 59, though it's seen in adults of all ages. The lifetime risk of developing melanoma is about 2%, or one in 50 people. According to the most recent NCI's SEER Cancer Statistics Review, the melanoma survival rate five years after diagnosis for all stages combined is 91%. If the disease is localized, then the five-year survival is 98%. Patients with regional spread to lymph nodes have a five-year survival rate of 62%. Those with distant, metastatic melanoma have a 16% survival rate at five years following diagnosis.

Risks and Causes

The highest risk factor for development of melanoma in adults is a persistently changed or changing mole. The medical term for mole is "melanocytic nevus." However, the absolute risk of a mole transforming into melanoma is very low. It's higher in older men than in women. One population-based study estimated the risk for a mole in a 20-year-old to transform to melanoma by age 80 to be about one in 3,000 for men, and one in 11,000 for women. Prior personal or family history of melanoma increases the risk. White people who are sensitive to the sun and those who have a history of excessive sun exposure are also at increased risk. However, people of color still get melanoma.

Signs and Symptoms

An enlarging, discolored skin lesion with irregular-shaped borders is the classic sign of melanoma. Everyone should perform routine surveys of their skin; a monthly basis works well. Any noticeable changes in the appearance or size of existing skin lesions should prompt evaluation by a dermatologist. The most common site for development of melanoma in women is the extremities, while for men it's the trunk. The upper back is a very common location. However, melanomas can develop almost anywhere, including between fingers and toes and under thick layers of hair on the head.

Diagnosis

Most patients are referred by their primary physician to a dermatologist, plastic surgeon, or general surgeon for biopsy of suspicious skin lesions. Sometimes, the diagnosis of melanoma cells under the microscope by a pathologist may be difficult due to their notorious ability to mimic the appearance of other tumors. There are several types of melanoma, but the treatment for each is quite similar. The superficial spreading type is the most common.

Staging

Laboratory evaluation generally includes complete blood count, serum chemistries, and lactate dehydrogenase (LDH). The AJCC TNM system is used for melanoma staging. It's based on the depth of tumor penetration in the skin and underlying tissue, the involvement of lymph nodes or satellite tumor nodules, and the presence and site of any metastatic spread. All of these factors may impact the patient's prognosis or outcome. Melanoma staging also includes the serum LDH level, since this marker was found to be prognostic for patients with stage IV disease. Patients with very high LDH levels had a five-year survival of approximately 20%, while those with normal LDH had a five-year survival of 50%. Other prognostic factors include the presence or absence of ulceration, as well as the mitotic (growth) rate of the tumor cells. The overall survival for patients five years following melanoma diagnosis, relative to the general population, is approximately 90% for stage I, 60% for stage II, 50% for stage III, and 10% for stage IV.

Treatment

The standard treatment for localized melanoma is wide surgical excision (removal) with at least 1-2 cm margins, depending upon tumor size and location. Most surgical oncologists who treat melanoma routinely will perform a sentinel lymph node (SLN) biopsy. This procedure involves injecting the tumor with blue dye and radioactive tracer, which guides the surgeon to the first site(s) of lymph node drainage for the primary tumor. If these lymph nodes are removed and contain no cancer, then the likelihood of cancer cells being left behind in other lymph nodes is quite low. On the other hand, if the SLN biopsy is positive for cancer cells, then the surgeon will usually perform a completion lymph node dissection (LND) to remove the remaining lymph node tissue in that region. In addition to removing more of the patient's tumor burden, the LND gives the team of cancer specialists further information that's often valuable in guiding treatment. A major RCT that enrolled over 1,200 patients with "intermediate-thickness" melanomas (between 1 and 4 mm thick) randomized half of the patients to immediate SLN biopsy and the others to no further surgery after removal of the primary tumor.

Patients who had cancer present in the SLN underwent completion LND. The trial confirmed that patients with cancer cells present in the SLN dissection had a worse survival than those with negative SLN (not too surprising). Perhaps more importantly, patients with positive SLN who underwent immediate LND had an improved five-year survival rate (72% versus 52%) compared to the group who had no initial lymph node evaluation or surgery.

The role for postoperative radiation therapy (RT) in the treatment of melanoma is limited. Patients with residual disease at the primary site after surgery, multiple lymph nodes involved with tumor, or extracapsular extension beyond the lymph nodes into the nearby tissues may benefit from postoperative RT to improve local control. The acute side effects of RT are site-dependent. In the head and neck region, acute skin redness and sore throat are the most common toxicities. One common RT regimen consists of five large doses or fractions delivered over two to two-and-a-half weeks. The total dose is moderate, 30 Gy. This regimen was shown to have a low risk of local or regional cancer recurrence in a group of patients treated for melanomas of the head and neck region. Occasionally more standard fractionation over four to seven weeks is utilized. Long-term side effects are uncommon, although fibrosis or scarring of soft tissue can occur, occasionally causing chronic stiffness or pain.

Systemic therapy for melanoma can be broken down into two main indications. Patients who have high-risk primary melanoma (thick, ulcerated, etc.) may benefit from postoperative systemic therapy. The main treatment in this situation is immunotherapy. Interferon alfa (IFN) and interleukin-2 (IL2) are both cytokines, a type of immunotherapy that's been used extensively over the past couple of decades for the treatment of patients with high-risk melanoma. Multiple RCTs testing IFN in this setting have shown a small benefit in decreasing the risk of cancer returning, sometimes even improving survival. The trials tested treatment durations ranging up to five years, but without significant benefit shown beyond about one year. A massive meta-analysis including 14 RCTs and over 8,000 patients (half of whom were randomized to treatment with IFN) showed a very small survival benefit to IFN, but no optimal dose or duration. The most common schedule for IFN currently is one month of high-dose, followed by one year of low-dose treatment. Many patients don't complete the full year of treatment, since most describe it as "like having the flu for a year." Severe fatigue and poor appetite are the main side effects.

The other main situation where systemic therapy is recommended is for patients with incurable, metastatic melanoma. The chemotherapy drug, dacarbazine, can be effective for these patients. The most common multidrug regimen includes cisplatin and vinblastine with dacarbazine (called CVD). A couple major RCTs have tested CVD chemotherapy with or without IFN and IL2, delivered either concurrently (at the same time) or sequentially (one after the other). Although there's a benefit to biochemotherapy (chemo plus IFN and IL2) in prolonging the time until the cancer progresses or grows, the improvement is only about two months. Side effects are worse with biochemotherapy than with CVD alone, and include severe fatigue, poor appetite, and decreased blood counts. Lastly, recently an exciting RCT was published using a new drug called ipilimumab for patients with metastatic melanoma that had progressed despite prior treatment. Ipilimumab is a type of monoclonal antibody (the "-mab" at the end of the word is the clue) that revs up the body's immune T cells to attack cancer cells. The trial revealed a significant survival benefit for the two groups of patients that received ipilimumab over the third group that didn't. Unfortunately, significant toxicity, including severe fatigue and GI issues, occurred in 10% to 15% of patients. There's a clear need to decrease the immune-related side effects of treatment for melanoma.

Dale's Melanoma Treatment and Outcome

After his biopsy, Dale was referred to a surgeon specializing in the treatment of melanomas. He underwent a wide local excision of the lesion on the back of his right shoulder, as well as a sentinel lymph node dissection in the right axilla (under the arm). On pathologic review, the melanoma invaded to a depth of 5 mm (about a quarter of an inch deep), though surgical margins were widely negative for tumor by 1.5 cm minimum.

There was evidence of cancer cells in one of three sentinel lymph nodes. A completion axillary node dissection revealed no evidence of cancer in 19 more lymph nodes. Dale was referred to a medical oncologist, who recommended interferon treatment. Dale declined this treatment. He had heard it "makes you feel like you have the flu for whole year," and wanted no part of it. He was seen regularly by his dermatologist and surgeon with no evidence of cancer recurrence for six years. At that time, however, he developed a severe right-sided headache, worse than he'd ever had in his life. An MRI of the brain revealed a 3 cm enhancing mass in the right frontal lobe worrisome for cancer. He was seen by a neurosurgeon and underwent resection of the mass confirming metastatic melanoma. Dale again refused any systemic treatment offered by his medical oncologist. He had consultation with a radiation oncologist, who discussed options of close observation versus RT to the brain in order to kill any residual microscopic cancer cells. Dale opted for close observation. It's only been eight months since his brain surgery, but he has no evidence of disease at this time.

MYELOMA

Norman's Story

Norm was a 72 year old retired accountant who never smoked in his life and was in reasonable health overall. He was an avid reader and chess player who enjoyed gourmet dining with his wife of 45 years. One day when his dog jumped up on him, excited about getting ready for a walk, Norm felt sudden pain in his back. His wife took him to the emergency department at the local hospital. There the doctor noticed Norm had severe tenderness in the lower thoracic spine, but no neurologic problems such as weakness or numbness of the arms or legs. A plain x-ray of the spine showed a fracture of the T10 vertebral body. He was admitted to the hospital to optimize pain control and for further evaluation. Norm underwent MRI of the spine that confirmed a fracture at T10 which appeared pathologic, not due to clear trauma. Blood tests revealed mildly low hemoglobin, normal creatinine (measure of kidney function), slightly elevated calcium, and a normal prostate specific antigen (PSA) level. A CT-guided biopsy of the T10 lesion revealed abnormal plasma cells in the bone consistent with likely myeloma. (To be continued….)

Myeloma is a type of "liquid tumor" similar to leukemia in that the majority of the cancer cells are in the blood and/or bone marrow. The abnormal cells in the case of myeloma are plasma cells, a part of the body's immune system. There will be approximately 20,000 patients diagnosed with myeloma, and 11,000 patients will die of their disease in the United States in 2010. The median age at diagnosis is 70 years old, and it's rarely diagnosed prior to age 45. The lifetime risk of being diagnosed with myeloma is 0.6%, or one in 160 people. Although it's rare to find localized disease, the five-year survival rate for this group of patients is 71%. More commonly, cancer cells are diffusely spread throughout the blood and bone marrow, and the overall myeloma survival rate at five years is 38%, according to the NCI's SEER database. Myeloma makes up 1% to 2% of all cancers. A precursor to myeloma, called monoclonal gammopathy of undetermined significance (MGUS), occurs in about 5% of the population over age 70. The rate of progression from MGUS to myeloma is just over 1% per year. MGUS may also transform to other malignant blood disorders.

Risks and Causes

Most patients have no clear risk factor for myeloma other than advanced age. Certainly, as mentioned above, a prior diagnosis of MGUS places patients at higher relative risk for developing myeloma subsequently. Black patients have a higher risk than whites, and men are at slightly higher risk than women. Patients with a positive family history of myeloma have an increased risk, although a family history is fairly uncommon.

Signs and Symptoms

Common presentations for patients with myeloma include generalized weakness or fatigue due to anemia and/or pain in the back, hips, or ribs due to direct bony involvement of those sites. Other patients develop recurrent infections since abnormal plasma cells leave little space in the bone marrow for production of normal immune cells. The body's immune system doesn't function as it should in this situation. Less commonly, patients present with hypercalcemia (a high calcium level in the blood) that may cause multiple symptoms including mental confusion, anorexia, nausea, vomiting, and abdominal and/or bone pain.

Diagnosis

There are several criteria that are required to make a multiple myeloma diagnosis. Laboratory evaluation should include complete blood count, a complete metabolic profile including kidney function and blood calcium levels, as well as the level of beta 2 microglobulin in the blood. Special tests to detect levels of myeloma in the blood serum and urine by protein electrophoresis, called SPEP and UPEP, should be performed. Bone marrow biopsies are standard to reveal the presence and amount of abnormal plasma cells in the marrow. For patients with lesions in the bone, diagnosis may be made by CT-guided biopsy.

Staging

Unlike most other cancers, the AJCC TNM system is not used for myeloma staging. Historically, the Durie-Salmon staging system has been used. This system is based on multiple factors, including blood levels of hemoglobin, calcium, and abnormal immunoglobulins (immune proteins); kidney function; and the presence and number of tumors in bones. The other common system utilized currently is the International staging system for myeloma. This system includes measurements of beta-2 microglobulin in the blood, since patients with low levels have been shown to have a significantly longer survival than those with high beta-2 microglobulin levels.

Treatment

Many patients with myeloma are asymptomatic (have no symptoms) and may not require treatment immediately. Since there's essentially no available cure for myeloma, the goal of treatment is to improve quality of life. If a patient has painful sites of bony metastasis, then a short course of palliative radiation therapy (RT) may be recommended. RT is generally delivered in low doses over a two-week course and has a 70% to 80% chance of improving pain. Treatment with a type of medication called bisphosphonates has been clearly shown to decrease patients' pain, decrease the risk of future fractures, and improve overall quality of life. A frequently prescribed bisphosphonate, pamidronate, is delivered by vein (IV) about once per month on an outpatient basis.

There are multiple systemic options for patients with myeloma. Symptomatic patients may be divided into two main categories: those who are eligible for high-dose chemotherapy with bone marrow transplantation (BMT; the minority) and those who are ineligible (the majority). In general, high-dose chemotherapy followed by BMT is reserved for younger patients in very good to excellent condition. For relatively young, healthy patients, a clear survival benefit has been shown in RCTs for this aggressive treatment over standard conventional dose chemotherapy. A couple of these RCTs showed that high-dose chemotherapy with BMT improved patients' survival by a full year or more, which is quite a difference for one treatment type over another. Currently, initial treatment regimens for patients prior to BMT include combinations of the steroid dexamethasone with thalidomide, lenalidomide, and bortezomib with or without thalidomide. Thalidomide and lenalidomide (a derivative of thalidomide) act by decreasing new blood vessel formation from tumors, thereby preventing their growth. Bortezomib is an example of a newer class of biologic agent called a proteosome inhibitor. A major trial from the Netherlands published early in 2010 revealed that incorporating thalidomide into initial treatment, called "induction," as well as after high-dose chemotherapy as "maintenance" therapy improved patients' outcomes. In the United States, lenalidomide is replacing thalidomide as maintenance treatment for patients with myeloma since it's generally better tolerated with less side effects.

The majority of patients with myeloma are too old or otherwise ineligible to receive high-dose chemotherapy with stem cell or bone marrow rescue (BMT). Standard chemotherapeutic agents that have been used to treat patients with myeloma include cyclophosphamide, doxorubicin, melphalan, and vincristine. Of these, the most commonly utilized is melphalan. For decades, it's generally been used in combination with prednisone. However, multiple RCTs of older patients who were not candidates for high-dose therapy have shown a clear benefit to the addition of either thalidomide or bortezomib over MP alone. A third common regimen used for the treatment of older patients is lenalidomide and dexamethasone. In fact, these two drugs are often prescribed for patients whose disease has returned after treatment with one of the other regimens. Common side effects of these medications include fatigue and decreased blood counts, sometimes causing a high risk of severe infection. Patients who receive thalidomide or lenalidomide are also at high risk for development of blood clots, so preventative blood thinners are often given to decrease this risk.

Norman's Myeloma Treatment and Outcome

Although he was in decent shape for his age, Norm couldn't tolerate high-dose chemotherapy with bone marrow transplant, according to his doctors. A two-week course of palliative external beam RT dramatically improved his back pain to where he could do what he wanted to do. He took only an occasional narcotic for pain before bed. His medical oncologist treated him with melphelan, prednisone, and thalidomide for several months. Norm got a good response and did well, without disease progression, for almost a year. However, his kidney function gradually began worsening, and he was becoming more anemic. He was tried on bortezomib, which kept things stable for a couple more months, before the disease progressed fairly rapidly. He developed a severe pneumonia, from which he didn't recover, about 18 months following his initial diagnosis. He died in the hospital with his wife by his side.

OVARIAN CANCER

Carol's Story

Carol was a 49-year-old middle-school teacher and avid tennis player. She had a history of prior surgery to remove her appendix and gallbladder but was otherwise very healthy. Over a period of about four months, she noticed that her belly seemed to be getting larger. Also, over the past month, she had started having vague pains on both sides of her pelvis that would come and go. She went to her gynecologist, who noticed mild tenderness on both sides during her pelvic exam but felt no masses. She sent Carol for an ultrasound that revealed a complex right ovarian mass. She underwent a CT scan of the abdomen and pelvis that confirmed the mass but showed no further abnormalities. Her primary gynecologist referred her to a gynecologic oncologist, who obtained blood tests, including a CA125 level that was very high. He recommended major surgery for what appeared to be an ovarian cancer. (To be continued....)

Ovarian cancer is the most deadly gynecologic malignancy in the United States, with an estimated 14,000 deaths expected to occur in 2010. It's also the second most common gynecologic cancer, with 22,000 women estimated to be diagnosed this year. The median age at diagnosis is 63. Younger women can also develop ovarian cancer. A woman's lifetime risk of developing this disease is about 1.5%, or one in 70 women. According to the most recent

NCI's SEER Cancer Statistics Review, the five-year ovarian cancer survival rate for all stages combined is 46%. If the disease is localized to the ovary (rare), then the five-year survival is 94%. Patients with regional spread to lymph nodes have a five-year survival rate of 73%. Those with metastatic ovarian cancer have a 29% survival rate at five years following diagnosis.

Risks and Causes

There's some evidence that women whose diet is high in fat may have an increased risk of this disease. Also, women who've never been pregnant or given birth (nulliparous) have a higher risk of developing ovarian cancer. Those who have taken hormone replacement therapy, particularly unopposed estrogen supplementation, also may be at increased risk. Women who carry mutations of the BRCA1 and BRCA2 genes have a risk of not only breast cancer but also ovarian cancer. Their risk of developing ovarian cancer is 15% to 45% with BRCA1 and about 10% with BRCA2 mutations. Fortunately, these mutations currently occur in a small portion of the general population. Women who have multiple close relatives with breast and/or ovarian cancer should strongly consider speaking with a genetic counselor about this type of testing.

Signs and Symptoms

Since the symptoms of ovarian cancer may be very slow in onset, women often attribute them to other causes. For instance, there are a multitude of potential reasons for the development of vague abdominal pain and/or an increase in abdominal girth or size. For these reasons, ovarian cancer is rarely diagnosed early. Occasionally, a complex cyst in the ovary may be seen incidentally during imaging for other causes in a patient who's completely asymptomatic (has no symptoms). This situation is usually favorable for the patient, since the disease may be diagnosed at an earlier stage.

Diagnosis

When an ovarian mass is felt on physical examination or seen on imaging, the patient should be referred by her primary physician or gynecologist to a gynecologic oncologist, a surgical specialist in the treatment of women's cancers. Often the pelvic examination or imaging findings are so consistent with a diagnosis of ovarian cancer that patients go directly to surgery. The proper surgery to treat ovarian cancer is an exploratory laparotomy with resection not only of the primary ovarian mass, but also of the uterus, fallopian tubes, and the other ovary. During surgery, washings of the pelvic and abdominal cavities with saline are also performed in order to detect any stray cancer cells. Lastly, removal of lymph nodes within the pelvis and para-aortic region is also part of the standard surgery. There are a couple of main types of ovarian cancer that are differentiated by the pathologist after viewing the cells under a microscope. Roughly 90% of patients are diagnosed with adenocarcinomas of epithelial (surface cell) origin. Another 5% have cancer of stromal (support) cells, and the other 5% have germ cell tumors. The remainder of the chapter will focus on epithelial ovarian cancer, the most common type.

Standard laboratory tests should be complete blood count, serum chemistries including kidney and liver function, and blood levels of a marker called CA125. This marker is elevated in approximately 85% of patients with ovarian cancer. However, as with most blood tests, the CA125 isn't 100% accurate. The level may be elevated with uterine cancer, as well as several benign (noncancerous) illnesses. When a patient does have ovarian or uterine cancer, the CA125 level may predict the burden of cancer cells existing throughout the body. In fact, it predicts ovarian cancer survival fairly well. CA125 is usually an excellent measure of how the cancer is responding to treatment.

Staging

Most patients have undergone ultrasound of the pelvis and/or CT scan prior to diagnosis and/or surgery. The historical ovarian cancer staging system that has been used is called the FIGO system. However, the AJCC TNM system is being more widely used. Early stage disease limited to the ovaries is rare. Advanced ovarian cancer with spread to lymph nodes and other parts of the abdomen is common. While metastatic ovarian cancer may be found in various parts of the abdomen and elsewhere in the body, the liver is a frequent site for distant spread.

Treatment

Patients with very early disease that's limited to one ovary, completely removed with negative surgical margins (no evidence of cancer cells at the edges of the surgical specimen), and of low grade may be treated with surgery alone, followed by close surveillance thereafter. Again, this situation is unfortunately quite rare. More commonly, extensive surgery is required that includes removal of the uterus, both ovaries, and fallopian tubes (TAH/BSO for total abdominal hysterectomy/ bilateral oophorectomy). Washings of the pelvis and abdominal cavities as well as extensive lymph node dissections in the pelvis and para-aortic regions are performed. Any sites suspicious for distant disease within the abdomen are usually removed if they can be resected safely. A "maximal debulking" that includes removal of all visible tumor nodules of 1 cm or larger improves patients' outcomes. When only microscopic cancer cells remain after surgery, then chemotherapy has a better chance of eliminating residual disease for a longer time. Patients who have residual, unresectable disease after surgery tend to fare poorly. Side effects of surgery for ovarian cancer include abdominal pain, risk of infection, and postoperative bowel problems, including a low chance of bowel obstruction or wound problems requiring reoperation.

Most patients with ovarian cancer require surgery followed by postoperative chemotherapy, usually for six full cycles or treatments. The standard regimen for ovarian cancer incorporates two drugs: carboplatin and paclitaxel. Initial RCTs revealed a benefit to cisplatin and paclitaxel over prior combinations. Then, a major RCT was completed that compared the combination of paclitaxel with either carboplatin or cisplatin. This trial revealed that carboplatin had the same survival but with less side effects and better ease of use than cisplatin. Carboplatin doesn't carry the same risk of damage to kidneys and hearing that cisplatin does, though it can decrease blood counts significantly. Multiple other IV chemotherapy regimens have been tested in the past, but none have proven superior. A couple of major RCTs have shown a benefit to delivery of cisplatin chemotherapy directly into the abdominal cavity rather than IV. This method, called intraperitoneal (IP) delivery, isn't widely prescribed throughout the United States due (at least in part) to its relative complexity compared to IV delivery. The common acute side effects of IV carboplatin and paclitaxel include fatigue, poor appetite, body aches, decreased blood counts with risk for infection, and a risk of nerve damage that may be permanent only in rare cases.

In the past, radiation treatment (RT) was delivered in low doses to the entire abdomen postoperatively for women with advanced cancer following maximal debulking of tumor. This whole abdominal RT improved outcomes in a major RCT. However, it's not commonly utilized today, since carboplatin and paclitaxel are fairly safe and effective treatments for the majority of patients. Palliative RT may offer significant reduction in pain and improvement in quality of life for patients with focal masses that aren't able to be removed surgically.

Carol's Ovarian Cancer Treatment and Outcome

Carol agreed to surgery. Her gynecologic oncologist performed a TAH/BSO with pelvic washings and a lymph node dissection. This surgery revealed an adenocarcinoma arising from the right ovary that also involved six of nine right and two of ten left pelvic lymph nodes, with multiple small deposits of tumor that had to be peeled off the fatty tissue in her abdomen. She had difficulty with a partial bowel obstruction postoperatively that resolved over several days. She then underwent chemotherapy with carboplatin and paclitaxel for six cycles, which she tolerated fairly well. Her CA125 level dropped to normal for over a year before it began to rise again. She received second line chemotherapy with topotecan, which she also tolerated well. She had good response for another nine months before her disease recurred. Third line chemotherapy kept her disease in check for another six months. When her disease returned this time, she was exhausted and had no further desire for more chemotherapy. Four months later, after further general decline, she opted for home hospice care.

Unfortunately, she had to be admitted to the hospital for a bowel obstruction six weeks later from which she did not recover. She died with her loving husband and two of her children at her hospital bedside.

PANCREATIC CANCER

Jerry's Story

Jerry was a 65-year-old man who had just retired from his position as regional sales manager of a national manufacturing company. He had a history of high blood pressure and chronic heartburn. He was a nonsmoker and drank alcohol only rarely. Jerry was very much looking forward to the rest and relaxation of his retirement. When he developed pain in his upper abdomen, he thought he might be getting a stomach ulcer. However, the pain had become more intense over three to four weeks and began radiating into his back. Over the past three months, he had noticed that he'd lost about 15 pounds. Ultimately, he went to his primary physician, whose exam revealed tenderness over the upper central abdomen but no palpable mass and no jaundice (yellow skin). Laboratory tests were normal except for levels of amylase and lipase enzymes in his blood that were slightly high. He had a CT scan which revealed a 5 x 3 cm mass in the head of the pancreas that appeared to be encasing the main artery nearby. He was referred to a gastroenterologist who performed an endoscopic retrograde cholangiopancreatogram (ERCP). Biopsy of the mass during the ERCP revealed an adenocarcinoma, pancreatic cancer. (To be continued....)

Cancer of the pancreas will be diagnosed in 43,000 patients in 2010 in the United States, and 37,000 patients will die of this disease. Despite being diagnosed much less frequently than some other cancers such as those of the breast and prostate, pancreatic cancer kills a similar number of people each year. It remains the fourth leading cause of cancer death. The median age at diagnosis is 72 years old, and it's rarely diagnosed in people younger than age 35. The lifetime risk of a pancreatic cancer diagnosis is 1.4%, or one in 72 people. According to the most recent NCI's SEER Cancer Statistics Review, the five-year survival following a diagnosis of pancreatic cancer is 6%. If the disease is localized, then the five-year survival is 22%. Patients with regional spread to lymph nodes have a five-year survival rate of 9%. Those with distant, metastatic pancreatic cancer have a 2% survival rate at five years following diagnosis.

Risks and Causes

The majority of patients are diagnosed without a clear major risk factor. It's more common as people age into their 60s and 70s. Pancreatic cancer is also more common in men than women and is diagnosed relatively more frequently in blacks than in whites. A widely recognized risk factor is a history of tobacco use, which may double or triple a person's risk. Chronic pancreatitis, or inflammation of the pancreas usually over years, also places people at increased risk for a pancreatic cancer diagnosis. People who have diabetes have a higher relative risk than the general population, although the absolute risk is small. Most patients with diabetes won't get pancreatic cancer. People who eat a high-fat diet long term also place themselves at increased risk. While not all of these risk factors can be modified (age and sex, for instance), a few of the others (smoking and diet) certainly can be.

Signs and Symptoms

Perhaps the most classic symptom of pancreatic cancer is upper abdominal pain radiating to the back. In general, however, pancreatic cancer symptoms depend upon whether the mass is located in the head, body, or tail of the organ. If a mass in the head of the pancreas (a common location for cancer) obstructs the biliary tree, then jaundice may result. Patients who develop jaundice may have yellow discoloration of the whites of their eyes or skin. They may also notice light-colored stools as well as dark "tea-colored" urine classically. Unexplained weight loss is very common. The amount of weight loss can be significant, sometimes more than 20 to 30 pounds, or a 10% to 20% decrease from baseline.

Diagnosis

Most patients who present with the above symptoms and/or signs undergo CT of the abdomen with contrast to evaluate the pancreas and bile ducts. If the radiologist sees a mass in the pancreas, biopsy under CT or ultrasound guidance may be performed. In other cases, patients are referred to a GI specialist for a procedure called an ERCP (as noted in Jerry's story above), during which pancreatic biopsies may also be performed. The vast majority of pancreatic cancers are aggressive adenocarcinomas, although low grade cancers are encountered occasionally. Metastasis to the pancreas from other primary types of cancer is a rare occurrence.

Staging

Standard laboratory evaluation includes complete blood count, serum chemistries, amylase and lipase levels (enzymes related to the pancreas), as well as CA 19-9 blood level. CA19-9 may serve as a marker of disease burden in the body. Like CA125 levels for ovarian cancer, the CA19-9 level in pancreatic cancer may be used as a measure of response to treatment if it's elevated initially. In addition to CT of the abdomen, patients may undergo endoscopic ultrasound (EUS) for further evaluation of the primary tumor and nearby lymph nodes.

Pancreatic cancer staging is based on the AJCC TNM system. Early stage cancers (those that are small in size, limited to the pancreas, and able to be removed surgically) are uncommon. In fact, only about 15% of patients are candidates for surgery at the time of the diagnosis. Most experts would say that surgery is the only potential for cure, but that even among those who have surgery, long-term survival is rare. Unfortunately, most patients present with locally advanced disease, where the pancreatic mass encases major blood vessels or regional lymph nodes are involved. Spread to distant sites at the time of diagnosis is very common. The most likely sites of metastasis are the liver and elsewhere in the abdomen. In addition to TNM staging, other prognostic factors that may be important for pancreatic cancer include CA19-9 level, presence or absence of tumor invasion into nearby lymphatic channels and nerves, and the amount of residual tumor left behind after surgery (in those who are candidates).

Treatment

For patients who have tumors that are able to be removed surgically and are in reasonable overall condition, the procedure that's performed is called a pancreaticoduodenectomy, also called a Whipple resection. This procedure usually involves removal of most of the pancreas, a portion of the stomach, the first portion of the small bowel called the duodenum, the gallbladder, and main part of the bile duct. Obviously, the Whipple procedure is a major surgery. In most expert oncologists' opinions, these procedures are best performed by surgeons who do them on a regular basis. What defines "regular" may be arguable, but a minimum of one case per month isn't an unreasonable expectation. Acute side effects of pacreaticoduodenectomy include risk of bleeding, infection, breakdown of the areas that were surgically sewn or stapled together, and a low but real risk of dying in the immediate postoperative period. Delayed emptying of the stomach after surgery is common, though this usually resolves quickly. Enzyme deficiencies and chronic bowel problems may also occur. Other variations of surgery, including those that have extended the amount of lymph node tissue removed, have not proven to be beneficial.

There's a clear role for postoperative gemcitabine chemotherapy for patients with locally advanced disease. The medication has also been shown to be quite effective for patients who have incurable, metastatic pancreatic cancer. The most common side effects of gemcitabine acutely include fatigue, poor appetite, nausea, vomiting, diarrhea, and decreased blood counts with risk of infection and/or bleeding. Rare but serious injury can occur to the kidneys, lungs, or liver. Postoperative chemoRT is more controversial. One RCT from Europe that was completed a few years ago called into question the benefit of postoperative chemoRT. It showed a decrease in survival for patients who received postoperative chemoRT compared to the group of patients that didn't receive it. However, there were major problems with the design and implementation of this trial. One major problem was that the prescribed RT dose was less than normally prescribed in the United States and incorporated a big break in the middle of treatment. In this situation, it's likely that most patients received the side effects of RT but none of the benefits. A few other studies have shown either no benefit or a small benefit to chemoRT postoperatively.

Unfortunately, the majority of patients with pancreatic cancer aren't able to have surgery, since their disease is usually diagnosed when it's inoperable. For most of these patients with unresectable pancreatic cancer, concurrent chemoRT is the standard treatment. It's been shown to significantly improve overall survival over RT alone. The RT is delivered five days per week over a five- to six-week course to a dose of 45-55 Gy, utilizing 3DCRT or IMRT (though clear benefit for the latter hasn't been proven). The concurrent chemotherapy is fluorouracil (5FU) most commonly, which is delivered IV through a continuous pump. Some medical oncologists substitute the oral chemotherapy pill, capecitabine, in place of 5FU since it has very similar effects and is usually easier for patients to take.

The most likely acute side effects of 5FU and capecitabine are fatigue, diarrhea, and irritation of the lining of the mouth. A rare but sometimes severe side effect of these medicines is severe scaling of the hands and feet, called hand-foot syndrome. Even more rarely, patients may develop significant heart damage, including potential heart attack. Common acute side effects of RT for pancreatic cancer include fatigue, nausea, and vomiting, though the latter two are generally well controlled (or prevented) with medication. Rarely, patients may develop severe bowel problems, including obstruction requiring surgery. These RT side effects are related to the organs that lie next to the pancreas, including the stomach, liver, and small bowel.

Jerry's Pancreatic Cancer Treatment and Outcome

After Jerry's ERCP, he was referred to a hepatobiliary surgeon who had performed many pancreatic cancer surgeries. He felt that the mass was surgically unresectable due to invasion of the tumor around a major artery that could not be removed. Therefore, he sent Jerry for consultations with both medical and radiation oncology. Those specialists recommended concurrent chemoRT, followed by gemcitabine chemotherapy. Jerry had some nausea and fatigue during his chemoRT. However, these symptoms resolved shortly after completion. He then received gemcitabine, which he tolerated very well, with only mild fatigue and anorexia. Restaging CT scans revealed initial shrinkage of the tumor, which then remained stable for nine months. A repeat scan at one year after treatment revealed multiple metastases in the liver. Jerry was offered enrollment on a clinical trial testing a promising new agent for the treatment of recurrent pancreatic cancer, but he declined. His general health deteriorated over the next two months, at which time his family agreed to home hospice care. He died three weeks later.

PROSTATE CANCER

James's Story

James was a 69-year-old African American male, a former history professor. He enjoyed sailing with his wife during his retirement. He had a history of high blood pressure and diabetes that was well controlled. His wife made sure that he saw his primary physician at least once per year. His PSA blood test levels had always been in the range of 2.5-3.0 ng/ml for over a decade. However, his most recent PSA was 3.8, up from 3.0 ng/ml one year prior. His doctor had already discussed the pros and cons of PSA testing with him in detail on several occasions over the years. Since his father died of metastatic prostate cancer at age 65, James wanted to be vigilant with PSA testing. His doctor referred him to a urologist, who performed a digital rectal exam (DRE), which was normal. He then performed a transrectal ultrasound with multiple biopsies of the prostate. Among the 12 biopsies of his 28-gram prostate gland, three of six from the left lobe revealed Gleason 6 adenocarcinoma, prostate cancer. (To be continued....)

Prostate cancer is the most commonly diagnosed cancer in men (other than nonmelanoma skin cancer). It's estimated to be diagnosed in 218,000 men in 2010 in the United States, and 32,000 men will die of the disease. The median age at diagnosis is 68 years old, and it's rarely diagnosed before age 40. The lifetime risk of a prostate cancer diagnosis is 16%, or one in six patients.

According to the most recent NCI's SEER Cancer Statistics Review, the prostate cancer five-year survival rate is 100%. This five-year survival rate is high for two main reasons. First, many prostate cancers are slow enough in their growth rate that even if they remained untreated, most men would be able to live with their disease for more than five years before the cancer metastasized (spread to other sites) and eventually killed them. Second, about 80% of prostate cancers are detected quite early, when the disease is still localized to the prostate. This group of patients has a high cure rate long term with any of the currently available standard treatments. On the other hand, for patients who are diagnosed when the tumor has already spread to other sites, the five-year survival rate is 31%, according to NCI's SEER statistics.

Risks and Causes

Any man who has a prostate is at risk for developing prostate cancer. A family history of the disease clearly increases a man's risk. It's more common with increasing age. In fact, some experts say that if all men lived to be 90-100 years old, most would have some degree of cancer in their prostates. Some black men tend to have more aggressive or advanced prostate cancer at earlier ages than white men. Lastly, many people find it surprising to hear that tobacco smoking also increases a man's risk for prostate cancer.

Signs and Symptoms

Since the widespread use of the prostate-specific antigen (PSA) blood test, most men present when they are asymptomatic (have no symptoms). Occasionally, patients will have urinary symptoms such as frequency, burning, or difficulty starting or maintaining their urinary stream. Even more rarely, men with very advanced disease may have pain in the low pelvis or low rectum due to mechanical pressure from a cancerous prostate that may become hard as a rock.

Diagnosis

Over the past two decades, most men have been diagnosed with prostate cancer based primarily on an elevated PSA blood test obtained by their primary doctor or urologist. When elevated beyond the normal levels, the PSA test should raise the suspicion of the presence of cancer cells in the prostate. However, PSA can also be elevated due to infection, inflammation, or with benign prostatic hypertrophy (BPH), an enlarged prostate that doesn't contain cancer. Roughly one out of every four men with an elevated PSA will be found to have prostate cancer. Probably just as important as the absolute PSA value is the rate of rise of the PSA level over time compared to prior values. This rate of rise, often referred to as PSA velocity, may serve as a good indicator of tumor biology. For instance, the top normal PSA level in the blood for a 60-year-old white man is about 4.0 nanograms per milliliter (ng/ml) of blood. However, most experts would be more concerned about the presence of aggressive or potentially metastatic prostate cancer in a patient whose PSA climbed from 1.5 to 3.9 ng/ml over the course of one year than in a patient whose PSA rose from 4.0 to 4.1 ng/ml.

Men suspected of having cancer in their prostates based on an abnormal PSA or DRE are sent to a urologist, a surgical specialist in the management of problems of the genitourinary (GU) tract. During an outpatient office procedure called a transrectal ultrasound (TRUS), the urologist places a probe through the patient's anus into the rectum in order to see the prostate. Multiple biopsy samples (usually between six and twelve) are taken from both lobes of the prostate. Cancer can't be seen with the naked eye in most cases, since it's microscopic. The biopsy samples are sent to a pathologist, a medical specialist who reviews them under a microscope.

The pathologist determines not only the absence or presence of prostate cancer cells, but also how aggressive the cells appear. This particular type of evaluation of prostate cancer cells results in a Gleason score (GS) which ranges from 2 to 10. The pathologist looks at the biopsy material under the microscope and determines how different the cancer cells are from normal prostate cells, giving a rank of 1 to 5 (with 5 being most abnormal) for the major pattern of the cancer. Then, the pathologist gives a second score of 1 to 5 for the minor pattern within the tumor. The two scores (of 1 to 5) are added together for the final score of 2-10. Extremely low grade scores of 2 to 5 are very rare. A GS of 6 or less indicates less aggressive disease, a GS of 7 is moderately aggressive, and a GS of 8 to 10 indicates highly aggressive cancer. In general, a higher GS is an indicator of an increased risk of extracapsular extension (ECE; microscopic cells being present in the tissue just outside the prostate gland), as well as a risk of cancer spread into the lymph nodes of the pelvis, or occasionally into distant sites such as the bones.

Staging

The AJCC TNM system is used for prostate cancer staging. A large proportion of patients have stage T1C disease, which means that there's no grossly palpable cancer that can be felt on DRE by the doctor. These cancers are generally diagnosed based solely on the basis of an elevated PSA blood test (followed by positive biopsy). All other things being equal, it's more favorable to be diagnosed with stage T1C disease. On the other end of the spectrum, if the physician feels gross evidence of cancer extending outside the prostate gland on DRE (stage T3 or T4), that situation is much less favorable for the patient's outcome.

For most men with prostate cancer, no further imaging is required, since the risk of cancer spread to other sites is quite low. However, for patients with very elevated PSA levels or those with high GS, imaging that includes CT of the pelvis and a bone scan is recommended for completion of prostate cancer staging. These scans may show gross evidence of cancer spread into the pelvis or bones (or other sites) that would change treatment recommendations. MRI of the prostate is often utilized to evaluate the presence or absence of ECE in patients who are considering surgery as primary treatment for their cancer. Prostate MRI should also be used routinely for external beam radiation therapy (RT) planning.

A system that divides patients into three risk groups has been developed that's based on three main pieces of information: clinical staging, including the DRE; the PSA level in the blood; and the pathologic GS. When evaluated together, these variables allow cancer specialists to predict with reasonable accuracy which patients have low, intermediate, or high risk of ECE, spread to lymph nodes in the pelvis, and/or metastasis to the bones or other distant sites in the body. Low-risk patients have either a small amount or no palpable disease on DRE, PSA of 10 or less, and a GS of less than 7. High-risk patients have disease that's grossly palpable outside the prostate on DRE, PSA greater than 20, or a GS of greater than 7. Intermediate-risk patients fall between the two extremes. There are other secondary factors that may predict for how aggressively a prostate cancer may behave, including the rate of rise of the PSA blood test over time, the number and extent of positive biopsies, and the presence or absence of tumor invasion around nerves (called perineural invasion) among others. Patient factors, including overall health and the presence of any major medical problems, play a large part in decision-making about treatment as well. However, the foundation for prostate cancer treatment recommendations is risk grouping.

Patients who are good candidates and desire surgical removal of their prostate also will have a pathologic stage for their cancer once it's removed. The pathologic staging for prostate cancer is based upon the findings of the pathologist who reviews the entire prostate specimen after surgical removal. This pathologic staging is the main indicator as to whether any further treatment is indicated, such as postoperative RT.

Treatment

LOW-RISK

Prostate cancer treatment is based on multiple factors, but predominantly upon risk group. For many patients with low-risk disease, close observation with regular monitoring of PSA levels and no immediate treatment (sometimes termed active surveillance) is an excellent option. In general, patients who are older and/or in poor health with a high risk of dying of other diseases within the 10 to 15 years following their prostate cancer diagnosis are poorly served by aggressive treatment. Sometimes this concept is difficult for patients in the United States to comprehend. They hear the word "cancer" and want it treated yesterday. In Europe, however, the mind-set must be quite different, since patients choose this option for low-risk disease quite frequently. Several major trials have revealed that not treating prostate cancer immediately is a reasonable option for men with low-risk disease. Most urologists recommend reevaluation with PSA in this setting more frequently than annually. A common schedule would be a repeat PSA test every three to six months. Men who are very elderly or ill and wouldn't ever want or qualify for treatment shouldn't have their PSA tested at all. This decision makes common sense.

There are multiple excellent treatment options for men with low-risk prostate cancer. These include radical prostatectomy, brachytherapy, and definitive external beam RT. Other treatments which are currently nonstandard or have less information available about long-term cure rates include cryotherapy (freezing the prostate tissue) and high-frequency ultrasound (HiFU). The following discussion focuses on local treatment options with long-term evidence for efficacy and side effects: prostatectomy, brachytherapy, and external beam RT.

Surgery to remove the prostate, radical prostatectomy, has undergone significant improvements over the past decade or two. The transition from the standard open surgical procedure to laparoscopic to robotic-assisted prostatectomy has brought improvements in patients' quality of life, particularly acutely. In the hands of skilled urologists experienced in laparoscopic and robotic prostatectomy, patients have major and minor complication rates of about 5% and 15%. They're usually discharged from the hospital in one to two days. It remains to be seen whether these procedures will improve cure rates versus prior forms of prostatectomy. However, with a baseline historical cure rate of more than 90% for patients with low-risk disease (from high-volume cancer centers), further improvement seems unlikely. For most men with low-risk and some with intermediate-risk disease, prostatectomy may be an excellent treatment choice.

Nevertheless, patients who opt for surgical treatment of their prostate cancer must be aware of the risks. In addition to the common surgical risks of bleeding and infection, side effects specific to prostatectomy include incontinence, which now normally lasts only a couple of months, as well as a high risk of permanent erectile dysfunction (ED). There have been a few major population-based studies of patient-reported side effects after prostatectomy. The first study, published in 1993, evaluated a sample of about 1,000 Medicare patients, so all were more than 65 years old, and about half were in their 70s. Fully 30% of patients reported wearing pads daily, and almost 90% reported being unable to have erections sufficient for intercourse after surgery. Urologists experienced with "nerve-sparing" prostatectomies who select their patients very well will argue that permanent ED is seen less frequently. The second report was based on almost 1,300 men ranging from 39 to 79 years old who underwent radical prostatectomy between 1994 and 1995. In this group, 56% of men were younger than 65. At 18 or more months after surgery, 8% of men were incontinent and 60% were impotent. The third report was a major study published in 2008. It included responses from more than 1200 patients who had chosen either prostatectomy or one of two radiation options (discussed below) for treatment of their prostate cancer. Among partners of men who opted for prostatectomy, 44% reported distress about erectile dysfunction. Urinary incontinence was worst at 2 months after surgery, but gradually improved thereafter, according to most patients. Long-term patient-reported outcomes after robotic prostatectomy are anxiously awaited.

Another excellent option for patients with low-risk disease is prostate brachytherapy ("brachy" is Greek for "short," meaning that radiation is delivered over a short distance). This type of internal RT involves the placement of multiple radioactive seeds into the prostate gland with the goal of eradicating cancer. There are two main forms of brachytherapy: high dose rate (HDR) and low dose rate (LDR). HDR brachytherapy involves temporary placement of radioactive sources that deliver high radiation dose over a short time into the prostate, generally in two to four different doses or fractions delivered in the radiation oncology clinic. LDR brachytherapy for prostate cancer is much more commonly performed throughout the United States than HDR treatment. LDR prostate brachytherapy involves permanent placement of radiation seeds that deliver a continuous low dose of radiation to the prostate. The remainder of the discussion about prostate brachytherapy will describe the LDR procedure in detail.

Men who are interested in brachytherapy for treatment of their low-risk prostate cancer initially undergo a TRUS for planning. This planning procedure is generally performed by a radiation oncologist, a cancer specialist trained in the use of radiation for medical purposes. After medication to aid in relaxation and minimize discomfort, with the patient lying on his back and his legs in stirrups, the ultrasound probe is inserted into the anus. Multiple images of the prostate are obtained and extensive measurements of the gland are made. When brachytherapy is used as the sole method of treatment, it's usually recommended for men with not only low-risk disease, but also medium to small prostate glands, in order to ensure that the entire gland can be treated with radiation seeds. If the patient is deemed a good candidate for brachytherapy after the planning TRUS, then the radiation oncologist and physicist create a plan to treat the entire prostate with a small margin around it, based on the particular size and shape of the patient's gland. At the time of the brachytherapy procedure in the operating room, a team approach is generally employed that includes the patient's urologist, radiation oncologist, and medical physicist. The LDR procedure is most often performed under general anesthesia on an outpatient basis and takes roughly one hour. The most common radioisotope used is iodine-125 (I-125), though some doctors use palladium or cesium in certain cases. For treatment of an average size prostate of about 30 grams with average strength I-125 seeds, about 70 to 90 seeds would be implanted. Each seed is about the size of a grain of rice. The seeds stay permanently, but the I-125 in the seeds decays or dissipates by 50% about every two months. So, after about 10-12 months, there's very little radiation left.

My colleagues and I have performed LDR brachytherapy procedures for more than 600 men with prostate cancer over the past decade. Patients generally tolerate the procedure very well, and those with low-risk disease in our practice have enjoyed a greater than 90% chance for cure thus far. Brachytherapy is also a very cost-effective method of treatment (for men who are candidates) relative to the alternatives. The most common side effects include frequency or burning with urination, most commonly lasting from one to eight weeks following the procedure. Because the prostate lies between the base of the bladder and the front of the rectum, potential side effects are related to both of these organs. While the majority of patients who have acute side effects will have them resolve completely within the first couple of months after treatment, 15 to 20% may report urinary irritation up to a year after treatment. About 5% to 10% of patients will develop painless rectal bleeding anywhere from 6 to 24 months following the procedure, which generally resolves on its own over a few months. My colleagues and I recommend a baseline colonoscopy for men prior to treatment, so that if they develop rectal bleeding following treatment, we'll know that symptoms are due to the brachytherapy (and will likely be short-lived) rather than from an undetected colon cancer. The risk of bleeding is highest in men who are on blood thinners, including aspirin. The risk of a severe side effect following prostate brachytherapy that would require surgery to repair is very low, about 1% to 2%. The risk of severe side effects tends to be worse in patients who have a history of other chronic illnesses, including vascular disease and diabetes.

In general, brachytherapy or "seeds" is an excellent treatment for men with low-risk disease who want to be aggressive (aren't comfortable with no immediate treatment), don't want the invasiveness or side effects of prostatectomy, and don't want to have to travel daily for two months to get standard external beam treatment. The cure rate is higher than 90% and the side-effect profile is reasonable, with a very low risk of severe injury. It remains to be seen whether brachytherapy alone or in combination with five weeks of external beam RT is better for men with intermediate-risk disease, but an RCT is ongoing to answer this question. Men with high-risk disease who desire seeds as part of their treatment should have them as a "boost" for delivery of high radiation dose to the prostate after five weeks of RT, and also long-term medications to starve the body of testosterone (to be discussed later).

External beam RT is most commonly delivered by a machine called a linear accelerator. It's a very reasonable and effective treatment for prostate cancer that's improved significantly over the past two decades. Most patients being treated today receive a type of fancy computerized treatment planning called intensity modulated radiation therapy (IMRT) over a roughly two-month course, with multiple small doses or fractions of RT delivered five days per week. IMRT allows radiation oncologists to deliver higher doses to target tissues, while minimizing the dose delivered to normal organs. In order to improve the daily accuracy of these treatments, image guidance (IGRT) is often utilized. While IGRT can be accomplished by several different methods, most frequently men will return to their urologist for placement of three markers into the prostate prior to RT planning. They then undergo immobilization of their pelvis in the radiation oncology clinic in a form-fitted mold that's shaped to their midsection and thighs, which minimizes the amount of overall body motion during treatment. Then, CT and MRI scans of the pelvis are obtained in the treatment position. The medical physicist or dosimetrist then fuses these two sets of images on the RT planning computer system. Next, the radiation oncologist uses the computer planning system to contour the prostate and any other target tissues as well as critical normal organs where RT dose should be minimized. In the case of prostate cancer treatment, these critical nearby organs include the bladder, rectum, and femoral heads (where the thigh bone inserts into the hip joint). Once the patient begins daily IGRT, the markers that have been placed by the urologist are visualized daily by the radiation therapy technologists and radiation oncologist. Even very small motions of the prostate (1 mm to 2 mm) can be accounted for on a daily basis, in order to ensure that the target tissues are central within the IMRT beams during the entire treatment course. As with surgery and brachytherapy for low-risk disease, cure rates at 10 years are about 85% to 90% following definitive IMRT/IGRT.

Toxicities of external beam RT are related to the nearby organs, since the prostate sits between the front of the rectum and the base of the bladder. Radiation can damage both cancer cells and normal cells, though cancer cells can't repair the damage to DNA in the cells as well as normal cells in general. Still, normal tissue can be hurt by radiation. Most large reports of RT side effects are from the era prior to IMRT and IGRT use. A survey of more than 600 Medicare patients was performed, similar to the one completed for patients who underwent prostatectomy. When compared to those who had surgery for their prostate cancer, men who were treated with RT had lower rates of requiring pads for incontinence (7% versus 32%) and lower rates of impotence (23% versus 56% for men less than 70 years old). However, they had more problems with bowel dysfunction (10% versus 4%). The 2008 study of patient reported outcomes (described above) also included patients treated with external beam RT. Roughly 10% of men reported some degree of GI distress up to one year after treatment. It should be noted that some of these patients were treated with 3DCRT while some were treated with more modern IMRT techniques.

INTERMEDIATE-RISK

Patients with intermediate-risk prostate cancer have a moderate chance of ECE (microscopic cancer cells extending outside the prostate capsule into the tissues nearby). While surgery or brachytherapy alone may result in long-term cure rates of 80%, there's a potential increased risk of microscopic cancer cells being left untreated in these patients with PSA of 10-20, GS of 7, or those with more extensive palpable cancer within the gland on DRE. External beam IMRT has a theoretical benefit of being able to treat these tissues around the prostate with a wider margin and less difficulty. However, no reasonable RCT has been completed that would allow men to decide among these different treatment options, unfortunately.

At this point, the topic of what's broadly been termed "hormone treatment" should be introduced. There are two main different types of systemic (nonlocal) therapy that kills prostate cancer cells throughout the body. These are hormones and chemotherapy. The latter will be discussed in the section on metastatic prostate cancer. Since the growth of most prostate cancer cells is fueled by testosterone, it's long been known that taking away testosterone dramatically slows or temporarily stops the progression of prostate cancer. Initially, removing testosterone was achieved by surgical removal of a man's testicles, a procedure called orchiectomy. However, as one would expect, this procedure has both physical and psychological consequences. It's also irreversible. For the past few decades, chemical castration has been the preferred method of decreasing testosterone, with two main types of medicines. The first and most commonly used group of medications for treatment of high risk and metastatic prostate cancer is called LHRH agonists. These drugs act on the master gland in the body, the pituitary. LHRH agonists act continuously on the gland, overstimulating it, ultimately resulting in a drop in testosterone to castrate levels (similar to orchiectomy, but reversible). These drugs are generally given as a subcutaneous (SQ; under the skin) injection in the belly or butt once every three or four months. The other class of anti-male hormones is anti-androgens. These medicines block testosterone receptors on cells and prevent testosterone from fueling cancer cells. They're sometimes used in conjunction with LHRH agonists in what's termed "total androgen blockade." Common anti-androgens include flutamide, bicalutamide, and nilutamide. Unlike LHRH agonists, these drugs are pills that are taken every day.

For patients with intermediate-risk disease, there's strong evidence that the addition of LHRH injections over six months provides a survival benefit versus EBRT alone when moderate RT doses of about 70 Gy are used. However, in modern practice, IMRT allows delivery of RT doses that exceed 75 Gy routinely with minimal risk of severe injury. The necessity of LHRH injections when delivered in conjunction with high-dose IMRT remains unproven. National studies by the Radiation Therapy Oncology Group (RTOG) are ongoing to answer this question. LHRH agonists have several important side effects including erectile dysfunction (ED, or impotence, at least temporarily), hot flashes, slight weight gain, tenderness of breast tissue, and occasionally achy joints. Long-term use increases risk of heart problems, most notably in men whose hearts are in poor condition at baseline.

Therefore, men with intermediate-risk prostate cancer currently have multiple reasonable options for treatment. Urologists and radiation oncologists often make their treatment recommendations based on additional factors besides risk group. These include the patient's age, overall condition, other medical illnesses, prostate gland size, and the number or percentage of biopsies positive. Those on the favorable end of intermediate-risk disease, with perhaps one factor such as GS 7 or PSA 10-20, may be treated similarly to low-risk disease and often cured with brachytherapy or prostatectomy or IMRT alone. Again, the role of LHRH agonists in this setting is currently uncertain. Selecting these patients correctly can be a difficult task for the doctor and/or an unsettling choice for the patient. There's another ongoing RCT which randomizes patients between brachytherapy alone versus five weeks of IMRT followed by brachytherapy boost. This trial led by the RTOG may answer an important question as to whether the addition of EBRT to brachytherapy decreases the risk of prostate cancer recurrence by killing microscopic cancer cells in the tissues just outside the prostate gland. Definitive IMRT/IGRT provides men with intermediate-risk disease long-term survival without return of their disease that may be equivalent to brachytherapy or surgery. IMRT is frequently chosen by men who prefer a less invasive treatment, as well as those who aren't candidates for the other two options.

HIGH-RISK

Men who have palpable cancer outside of the prostate on DRE, a PSA higher than 20, or a GS of 8-10 are considered to have high-risk disease. In addition to a high risk of cancer cells extending outside the capsule of the prostate (ECE), these men have a moderate to high-risk of microscopic cancer cells being present in pelvic lymph nodes and potentially even in distant, metastatic sites such as the bones. These patients should all undergo CT or MRI of the pelvis as well as a bone scan to exclude gross evidence of distant metastases at the time of diagnosis.

In the opinion of most cancer experts, men with high-risk disease are poorly served by treatment with surgery or brachytherapy alone. The risk of leaving microscopic cancer cells behind with these procedures is exceedingly high. Patients who fail initial treatment may subsequently require further local and systemic treatments, and ultimately have a high risk of dying of metastatic prostate cancer. There are clear survival benefits to long-term LHRH use for men with high-risk disease who are treated with RT. The optimal local treatment option for most high-risk patients is definitive IMRT encompassing the prostate and a portion of the glands above the prostate called the seminal vesicles, at minimum. IMRT/IGRT may often include treatment of pelvic lymph nodes to a moderate dose of radiation, in order to kill microscopic cancer cells that may have spread there. An alternative local treatment choice is a combination of five weeks of IMRT followed or preceded by brachytherapy. Experts who favor this approach like the increased RT dose that's delivered to the prostate by the seeds, but opponents argue that the risk of side effects with combination treatment is higher than with IMRT/IGRT alone. Men with high-risk disease most commonly receive LHRH injections for a total of two to three years, based on major RCTs that revealed a survival benefit with that duration of treatment over RT alone.

POSTPROSTATECTOMY

When urologists select their patients for surgery well preoperatively (as the best urologists usually do), only about 10% to 15% of patients will have their cancer return. In this subset of patients, occasionally cancer cells are left behind at the surgical margin. In other instances, despite having a low PSA, no evidence of palpable cancer outside the gland on DRE, and a low GS preoperatively, pathologists may find microscopic ECE or tumor invasion into the adjacent seminal vesicles. Patients with these findings, as well as most men who develop a slowly rising PSA following surgery, will require postoperative RT for improved chance of survival. There's rarely good reason for a man with a high-risk prostate cancer to be subjected to a prostatectomy, since most men with stage T3-4 disease, PSA higher than 20 ng/ml, or GS 8-10 will require postoperative RT. These unfortunate men are subjected to the side effects of both treatments, but without clear benefit from their surgery.

Data indicate that postoperative IMRT should begin soon after surgery. Recent RCTs have confirmed decreased risk of cancer recurrence and one trial showed an overall survival benefit to immediate postoperative RT. Most radiation oncologists recommend initiation of IMRT once urinary continence has been restored, or at least shows no signs of further improvement following surgery. Although it's uncommon for IMRT to cause incontinence by itself, it's common for RT to halt improvement following prostatectomy. A recent report revealed that IMRT delivered after nerve-sparing prostatectomy had no negative effect on erectile function in patients who were potent after surgery.

METASTATIC

A minority of patients with initially localized prostate cancer will have their disease return in distant sites in the body following local treatment with radical prostatectomy, brachytherapy, or definitive IMRT. Other patients may have cancer that's already metastasized (spread) to distant sites at the time of their diagnosis. For these groups of patients, the primary method of treatment is "hormone therapy," as defined above in the section on intermediate-risk disease.

Of the two main types of medications, LHRH agonists have the most potent effects on decreasing testosterone rapidly. However, urologists will often also add oral anti-androgen pills to LHRH agonists for total androgen blockade (TAB). Depending upon the aggressiveness of the cancer cells, these medications can kill a large proportion of cancer cells and prevent the disease from progressing for an average of one to three years. Unfortunately, these treatments for patients with metastatic prostate cancer aren't curative. The LHRH or TAB kills only that portion of cancer cells which depends upon male hormones to grow. Unfortunately, after some time, the other portion of cancer cells that are independent of the male hormones begins to grow more rapidly. In general, repeat PSA blood level testing is the most accurate way to assess disease response to the hormonal therapy. At the time when the disease progresses on TAB, it's termed "hormone-resistant" or "castration-resistant" prostate cancer. Common side effects of LHRH agonists or TAB include hot flashes, weight gain of 5-10 pounds, gynecomastia (swelling with or without discomfort of the breast tissue; most common with long-term treatment), fatigue and joint aches.

In patients whose disease has become hormone-refractory or castration-resistant (no longer responds to TAB), the most common next treatment is chemotherapy. Docetaxel has reasonable activity against prostate cancer and is often the initial chemotherapy drug recommended by medical oncologists. It's been shown to prolong survival in men with castration-resistant prostate cancer. Mitoxantrone is another chemotherapy agent that can also be effective. The average life expectancy for men in this situation is about 12 to 22 months. Side effects of these agents include decreased blood counts, body aches, fatigue, poor appetite, and occasional numbness or nerve problems that may become chronic.

Lastly, a recently reported major RCT revealed a benefit to immunotherapy for patients with castration-resistant prostate cancer. The trial tested a drug called sipuleucel-T, a type of vaccine that's used for treatment rather than prevention of cancer. It's made from patients' own immune cells combined with a special protein that contains a prostate targeting agent as well as factors that stimulate and activate the immune system. In this RCT, investigators randomized men to receive the vaccine (once every 2 weeks for a total of 3 infusions) versus placebo. Only men with GS of 2-7 and no symptoms of their disease were eligible. In order to participate, the men also could not have received any chemotherapy, RT, bisphosphonates or steroid therapy within the prior month. Therefore, these patients were in better shape than most men with castration-resistant prostate cancer. Nevertheless, the group treated with sipuleucel lived an average of four months longer (26 versus 22 months) and their chance of being alive at three years after treatment was 9% higher than the group that received placebo.

BONE METASTASES

Although prostate cancer can metastasize to various sites in the body, the most common distant site of spread is to the bones. Patients may receive a benefit from a regular injection of a type of medication called bisphosphonates. These medicines are generally delivered by IV injection once every three to four weeks and have been shown to decrease the risk of future fractures as well as decrease bone pain. Palliative external beam RT to focal sites of painful bony metastases results in a 75% chance of decrease in pain. Although life is not extended, quality of life can be dramatically improved. The course of palliative RT is usually short, often two weeks or less. Side effects are dependent upon the site being treated, though they are generally minimal for treatment of small areas with no adjacent bowel or internal organs nearby. Another type of radiation called samarium-153 may also be delivered by IV injection in order to stabilize disease within the bones and decrease pain. Samarium is very effective treatment for metastatic prostate cancer that's spread diffusely to multiple bones. It's often used when disease is too extensive for external beam RT to be practical. The main side effect of samarium is a decrease in blood counts which is usually temporary.

James's Prostate Cancer Treatment and Outcome

Since James had a negative DRE (stage T1C), a PSA lower than 10, and a GS of 6, his disease was considered low risk. He was in reasonable health and had a medium-sized prostate gland at 28 grams. Therefore, he had essentially all options open to him. His urologist discussed risks and benefits of surgery, brachytherapy seeds, IMRT/IGRT, and active surveillance with no immediate treatment. James knew what prostate cancer had done to his father and was not comfortable with active surveillance. Two of his friends "had the seeds and they did great!" His urologist referred him to a radiation oncologist, who again explained all of his options, including the brachytherapy procedure, in great detail. He reviewed the 90% cure rate for men with low-risk disease, as well as potential side effects, including increased frequency or pain with urination for several months after the treatment, the risk of rectal bleeding or discomfort, and the 1% to 2% risk of severe injury to the rectum or bladder. James agreed to proceed and underwent a planning TRUS in the radiation oncology clinic, followed by brachytherapy on an outpatient basis at the local community hospital.

His urologist, radiation oncologist, and medical physicist worked together as a team for the procedure. The placement of the seeds looked excellent on the day of brachytherapy as well as on CT scan of the pelvis one month later. James had to get up about three times per night to urinate and had mild discomfort for about two months after the procedure, but these symptoms subsided soon thereafter. His PSA went from 3.8 ng/ml before the treatment down to 0.7 ng/ml by three months after seed placement. Subsequent PSA values decreased to a low of 0.2 ng/ml, where they have hovered for the past seven years. He remains without evidence of prostate cancer and is thoroughly enjoying his retirement.

SKIN CANCER, NONMELANOMA AND BETTY'S STORY

Betty's Story

Betty was a 64-year-old retired administrative assistant who loved to read and spend time at the beach. Unfortunately, she spent lots of time in the sun as a child without the benefit of sunscreen, and she rarely wore a hat to protect her face. She noticed a red round nodule with a shallow center arising over her left cheek over the period of three to four months. When she showed it to her dermatologist, her examination revealed a 1.5 cm (0.5 inch) nodular lesion with pearly raised borders, which she felt was classic for a basal cell carcinoma, nonmelanoma skin cancer. (To be continued....)

Nonmelanoma skin cancer is a broad term that refers to all cancers of the skin other than melanoma. However, in practical terms, skin cancer specialists usually equate the term with two main types of skin cancer: squamous cell (SCC) and basal cell carcinomas (BCC). By far the most common cancers in the United States, nonmelanoma skin cancers are diagnosed in over a million patients per year. The lifetime risk of developing one of these tumors is about 20%, or one in five people. Fortunately, among this massive number of patients, very few people die as a result of their skin cancer.

Risks and Causes

Sun exposure is the predominant risk factor for over 90% of those with a nonmelanoma skin cancer diagnosis. People who are fair-skinned and/or have an increased sensitivity to the sun have an increased risk for developing skin cancer relative to others in the general population. These risk factors can clearly be modified. Regular use of sunscreen and, believe it or not, consumption of a low-fat diet have both been shown to decrease the risk of solar (also called actinic) keratoses. By preventing these lesions that are cancer precursors (precancers), people can decrease their risk of skin cancers as well. One RCT revealed that regular sunscreen use decreased the risk of future SCC, though it wasn't as helpful for preventing BCC. A personal history of skin cancer is a strong predictor of future cancers. Patients whose immune system is suppressed due to other diseases or medications are also at significantly increased risk for these types of skin cancer. Lastly, patients who receive radiation have a small increased risk of developing BCC, but not SCC, according to a large study published by the Skin Cancer Prevention Study Group.

Signs and Symptoms

Many people are unaware of what skin cancers look like. Many folks worry at every new freckle or bump. Others, believe it or not, will wait until a grapefruit-sized mass is hanging off their head before they seek medical attention. There are many skin lesions that develop with aging. The vast majority of these are benign. In general, though, people who notice a new skin lesion that doesn't go away after a couple of weeks should pay a visit to their primary physician. A referral to a dermatologist may be recommended. Classically, BCCs appear somewhat nodular with "raised pearly" edges or borders. SCCs can form small nodules or may appear as scaly red spots that persist for weeks or months. Most nonmelanoma skin cancers don't cause a marked change in skin color otherwise and, if found early, aren't overly large. Only rarely do they grow rapidly.

Diagnosis

A skin specialist such as a dermatologist or plastic surgeon may remove part or all of a lesion as a biopsy to determine whether it's benign or malignant. Usually a pathologist will examine the biopsy to determine whether cancer is present as well as the type. Some dermatologic surgeons will perform their own pathology review of the biopsies that they perform to diagnose skin cancer.

Staging

The AJCC TNM system is used to stage skin cancers including SCC, BCC, and other less-common types. Imaging with CT or MRI may be recommended if the lesion is very advanced or in a critical location, to evaluate for possible tumor invasion deeper than the skin. MRI is the preferred method to check if a skin cancer has invaded nerves.

Treatment

For very early or in situ (pre-invasive) cancers, topical treatment may provide good local tumor control. One RCT from Scotland tested three different conservative, nonsurgical treatments: cryotherapy (freezing), topical fluorouracil chemotherapy, and photodynamic therapy (PDT) with topical methyl aminolevulinate. This trial revealed that PDT was superior to the other two methods, and cosmetic appearance was rated good to excellent by 94% of patients.

For most skin cancers, however, surgery is the treatment of choice. If the cancer is large, then the dermatologist may call upon a plastic surgeon for assistance. A special type of surgery called Mohs surgery may be recommended in many cases. During this procedure, the dermatologic surgeon removes a skin cancer in multiple thin layers, going deeper with each resection, and inspecting each specimen under the microscope until negative surgical margins (no tumor cells remaining at the edge) are obtained.

For tumors in extremely difficult locations such as the central part of the face, radiation therapy (RT) is often the treatment of choice. RT is most frequently recommended if/when surgical removal of the cancer would be disfiguring, or for patients who wouldn't tolerate surgery. In general, surgery alone is curative for patients with early stage skin cancer in more than 90% of cases. Similarly, for patients with early SCCs and BCCs in difficult locations, RT cures rates exceed 90%. Multiple series in the medical literature indicate that small tumors less than 2 cm (about an inch) in size are controlled 95% of the time by RT, whereas tumors larger than 5 cm are controlled less than 50% of the time. Tumors that invade cartilage, bone, or nearby nerves have a slightly higher chance of returning after treatment. Patients who are unfortunate enough to have nerve invasion that causes symptoms also have about a 50% control rate. It's important to see a dermatologist long before symptoms occur.

Cosmetic results with standard or Mohs surgery are usually rated good to excellent by patients. With RT, cosmetic results often depend on tumor size, which dictates the size of the radiation field. In one large RT series from the United States, cosmesis was described as good to excellent by more than 90% of patients. On the other hand, in a European RCT of surgery versus RT, patients and doctors felt that RT was inferior cosmetically. It should be noted, however, that RT techniques may differ dramatically between institutions.

As a rule, BCCs don't spread to regional lymph nodes, while SCCs often do, particularly when they're larger. In those cases, surgeons may perform a sentinel lymph node procedure to ensure that no microscopic cancer cells have spread, similar to the process for patients with melanoma. This procedure involves injecting dye and radioactive tracer into and around the skin cancer, then tracking with both methods into one or more adjacent lymph nodes which are then surgically removed. If the sentinel lymph nodes are negative, then the risk of other remaining lymph nodes being malignant is less than 5%.

Among patients who undergo surgical resection of their cancers, indications for postoperative RT include positive surgical margins, as well as lymphatic, vascular, and/or perineural invasion (cancer cells involving lymph vessels, blood vessels, or nerves adjacent to the tumor). For SCCs that have spread to multiple lymph nodes or extended beyond the lymph node capsule into nearby tissues, some oncologists recommend postoperative treatment with concurrent chemoRT. Although there are no major RCTs that support the use of chemoRT for skin cancer specifically, several major trials have shown benefits for postoperative chemoRT over RT alone for patients with SCC of the head and neck region. Many cancer specialists cite these trials as evidence that chemoRT should be used to treat very advanced SCC of the skin postoperatively.

Betty's Skin Cancer Treatment and Outcome

Betty's dermatologist referred her to a dermatologic surgeon who specialized in Mohs surgery since the lesion was in a difficult spot on her left cheek just beneath her lower eyelid. The surgeon removed the lesion using the Mohs technique, which confirmed basal cell cancer. She was able to remove the cancer with negative surgical margins and close the wound without need for plastic surgery. Betty had no evidence of tumor recurrence on her cheek, though she did develop several other nonmelanoma skin cancers over the next several years which were treated by her dermatologist without difficulty. One tumor between her lower left eyelid and her nose was treated with a four-week course of RT and cured, with an excellent cosmetic result also. Betty died of a presumed sudden heart attack in her sleep nine years later.

STOMACH CANCER

Frank's Story

Frank was a 72-year-old retired businessman. He enjoyed life fully, but his greatest pleasures were watching sports and eating good food. He had a history of high blood pressure, high cholesterol, and chronic heartburn, as well as prior surgery for a stomach ulcer many years ago. When he began to have pain in his upper abdomen, he feared that he had another stomach ulcer. Then, he started to notice changes in his bowels with what appeared to be dark blood in the toilet. He also felt much weaker and had lost about 10 pounds over the prior four to six weeks. He went to his primary doctor, whose examination revealed Frank to be pale, with tenderness over the upper central abdomen. Laboratory evaluation revealed his hemoglobin level (protein in blood that carries oxygen) to be 7 g/dl, about half of the normal level. Frank was admitted to the hospital and received a transfusion of blood, which made him feel better immediately. He was seen by a gastrointestinal (GI) diseases specialist, who performed an esophagogastroduodenoscopy (EGD), which revealed a 5 x 3 cm ulcer in the body of the stomach. Biopsy of the ulcer revealed an adenocarcinoma, stomach cancer. (To be continued....)

The numbers of patients diagnosed with stomach cancer (also called gastric cancer) vary greatly by geographic region across the world. In the United States, it's estimated that 21,000 patients will be diagnosed and 11,000 patients will die of the disease in 2010. There are some discrepancies in this regard depending on the source, since cancers that develop at the junction of the esophagus and the stomach ("GE junction") are sometimes grouped with cancers of the stomach, and sometimes with those of the esophagus. The latter grouping is the current AJCC recommendation. The median age for diagnosis of stomach cancer is 71, and it's rarely diagnosed before age 35. The lifetime risk of developing cancer of the stomach is about 0.9%, or one in 110 people. According to the most recent NCI's SEER Cancer Statistics Review, the five-year survival for stomach cancer, relative to the general population, for all stages combined is 26%. If the disease is localized, then the five-year survival is 63%. Patients with regional spread to lymph nodes have a five-year survival rate of 27%. Those with metastatic stomach cancer have a 3% survival rate at five years following diagnosis.

Risks and Causes

Patients with a history of prior gastric infection with the bacteria *Helicobacter pylori* are known to be at increased risk for a stomach cancer diagnosis. There's evidence that elimination of the infection decreases the risk of stomach cancer. Patients who've had prior major stomach surgery, as well as those with a history of diseases called chronic atrophic gastritis and pernicious anemia, are at increased risk.

Signs and Symptoms

Classic symptoms of stomach cancer include central upper abdominal pain, unexplained weight loss, and sometimes extreme fatigue due to blood loss. Patients with cancers of the GE junction may also develop dysphagia (food sticking during swallowing) or odynophagia (pain during swallowing). It may be difficult at first for the patient or primary doctor to differentiate between signs and symptoms of a possible stomach ulcer, which is very common, versus the less common but more life-threatening diagnosis of stomach cancer.

Diagnosis

In patients who present with the above symptoms and/or signs on physical exam, laboratory evaluation should include a complete blood count and complete metabolic profile, including tests of liver and kidney function, carcinoembryonic antigen (CEA) level, and alkaline phosphatase. The CEA level, which is commonly used as a marker for colorectal cancer, may also be elevated with stomach cancer in 15% to 20% of cases, especially if advanced disease is present. Once the diagnosis of a stomach ulcer or stomach cancer is suspected, a referral should be made to a gastroenterologist, a medical specialist in the treatment of diseases of the gastrointestinal tract. This doctor may perform an EGD (as in Frank's story above), also called an upper endoscopy. The procedure involves placement of a fiberoptic scope through the nose and throat, in order to look directly at the lining of the upper gastrointestinal (GI) tract, mainly the esophagus and stomach. Biopsy of any suspicious areas should be performed. Approximately 90% of stomach cancers are of the common glandular type, called adenocarcinomas. Occasionally patients will develop lymphomas of the stomach. Other subtypes are fairly rare.

Staging

After the EGD that provides both diagnosis and staging information, patients should have CT of the chest and abdomen, as well as consideration for bone scan if the cancer appears to be more advanced. PET/CT can be substituted for those two tests and may also be used for restaging postoperatively, in order to guide further treatment recommendations. Endoscopic ultrasound (EUS) is often performed at major cancer centers. This procedure provides additional information, including depth of tumor penetration into the GE junction or stomach wall, as well as potential enlarged lymph nodes that may be biopsied. Early stage disease is limited to stomach lining and muscle. Advanced stage disease includes deep tumor penetration through the stomach wall and/or involving nearby lymph nodes. Patients who present with metastatic stomach cancer to the liver or other organs are considered to have stage IV disease, generally incurable.

Treatment

Fortunate patients who have their gastric cancer diagnosed at an early stage may undergo surgery alone. A procedure called a subtotal gastrectomy (SG) usually removes about 70% to 80% of the stomach, the omentum (the fatty, drapelike lining in the abdomen that overlies the stomach), and a portion of the duodenum (first section of the small bowel). According to major RCTs, the 50% to 60% survival rate for patients undergoing SG was essentially the same as patients undergoing total gastrectomy (removal of the entire stomach). Recent trials have shown that laparoscopic SG has the same cancer control rate as the open SG procedure, but with less blood loss and earlier discharge from the hospital for most patients. A major area of controversy has been the extent of surgical removal of lymph nodes near the stomach. The most recent trials indicate that removal of all of the regional lymph nodes near the stomach (called an extended lymphadenectomy) is indicated, but removal of lymph nodes near the aorta in the back of the abdomen doesn't improve patients' survival.

Patients who have locally advanced disease often require treatment in addition to surgery for the best possible outcome. Preoperative or postoperative treatment for stomach cancer may include chemotherapy and/or RT. Two major RCTs have shown a benefit to chemotherapy and concurrent chemoRT. The first trial included over 500 patients and was performed in multiple major cancer centers in the United States. It revealed an improvement in survival for patients who received postoperative chemoRT with fluorouracil, leucovorin, and RT to a dose of 45 Gy, versus those who were treated with surgery alone. At three years after treatment, 50% of patients were alive versus 41% in the group that didn't receive chemoRT. Many major cancer centers now treat patients with advanced gastric cancer with surgery and postoperative chemoRT according to this intergroup trial. However, patients with advanced cancer of the GE junction may receive chemoRT preoperatively. A major benefit of preoperative over postoperative RT includes potentially decreased RT field size, which may result in treatment of less normal small bowel and, therefore, fewer side effects.

The second trial, which also included about 500 patients but was performed in Europe, revealed a survival benefit to patients who received both preoperative and postoperative chemotherapy (no RT) over those that received surgery alone. The chemotherapy regimen included epirubicin, cisplatin, and fluorouracil (called ECF). In the trial, patients received three preoperative and three postoperative cycles. At five years after treatment, 36% of patients were alive in the chemotherapy group versus 23% of patients in the group treated with surgery alone. In several other recent trials testing postoperative chemotherapy, other medicines that have shown to be beneficial include capecitabine, oxaliplatin, and a drug called S-1, which is in the class of drugs called fluoropyrimidines.

In addition to the common surgical risks of bleeding and infection, acute side effects of surgery for stomach cancer include nausea, vomiting, diarrhea, and the risk of dumping syndrome, which is when undigested stomach contents reach the intestine, causing discomfort and bowel urgency. Patients who undergo SG also have a very small risk of developing a leak at the site where the bowel was sewn or stapled together, abscess (pocket of infection) around the pancreas, or fistula (hole between organs). RT to the stomach and nearby lymph nodes may cause fatigue, anorexia, nausea, vomiting, and bowel irritation. Severe inflammation of the bowel called enteritis is much less common. Common acute chemotherapy side effects with fluorouracial-based regimens include fatigue, poor appetite, diarrhea, and sometimes nausea. Uncommon side effects include hand-foot syndrome and rare severe damage to the heart. When patients are given preventative anti-nausea medication and are counseled regarding proper nutrition habits during chemoRT, they are generally able to complete treatment with a very low risk of serious side effects.

Frank's Stomach Cancer Treatment and Outcome

Frank's GI specialist referred him to a surgeon, who recommended a subtotal gastrectomy. He sent him for a CT scan of the chest and abdomen which revealed thickening of the stomach wall with several enlarged lymph nodes nearby, but no evidence of distant metastases. Frank underwent this major surgery, which revealed a 5 x 5 cm tumor extending through the stomach wall, with involvement of five out of 12 nearby lymph nodes.

His surgeon sent him for consultation with both a radiation and a medical oncologist, who recommended postoperative chemoRT. Frank underwent the five-week course with moderate nausea, but significant anorexia and severe fatigue. He lost another 20 pounds during chemoRT, down from a pretreatment weight of 195 pounds. It took two more months to recover, and his doctors recommended no further treatment since he was quite debilitated. He developed pneumonia three months later. Frank had already decided upon comfort care only, so he did not want to be admitted to the hospital. He died at home with his son at his bedside.

THYROID CANCER

Peggy's Story

Peggy was a 52-year-old restaurant hostess who had a thriving side business as a party planner. She had a history of severe arthritis in her hands and borderline high blood pressure, but was in otherwise good health. She went to her doctor for an annual check-up and was found to have a small lump on the right side of her midneck. Her blood tests showed that her level of thyroid hormone was slightly low. Her doctor referred her for an ultrasound of her thyroid and neck, which revealed a solid nodule in the right lobe of her thyroid, as well as an adjacent enlarged lymph node. Fine needle aspiration of the thyroid nodule revealed malignant cells consistent with thyroid cancer. (To be continued....)

The thyroid gland in the neck plays a major role in the body's metabolism. As people age, the risk of developing cancer in the gland increases. In the United States in 2010, it's estimated that 45,000 patients will be diagnosed, while 1,700 will die of the disease. Thyroid cancer is much more common in women (34,000 cases per year) than in men (11,000 cases per year). The median age at diagnosis is 48, and it's rarely diagnosed before age 20. The lifetime risk of a thyroid cancer diagnosis is about 0.9%, or one in 110 people. The overall survival for thyroid cancer five years after diagnosis for all stages combined is 97%, according to NCI's SEER statistics. Patients who have localized disease (the majority) have a five-year survival rate of 100%. Those who are diagnosed with metastatic disease still have a 58% five-year survival.

Risks and Causes

Radiation exposure is the most well-known risk factor for the development of thyroid cancer. However, the majority of patients who are diagnosed have no clear known risk factor. Females are about three times as likely to develop thyroid cancer as males.

Signs and Symptoms

The majority of patients are asymptomatic (have no symptoms). About 75% of patients diagnosed with thyroid cancer present to their doctor with a neck mass. Others are found to have a mass palpable on routine physical examination by their general doctor. About 25% of patients will report dysphagia, the sensation of food sticking when they swallow. Hoarseness or other voice changes can occur. Difficulty breathing occurs rarely with advanced or aggressive disease.

Diagnosis

Usually an ultrasound of the neck is obtained to evaluate any lumps felt in the thyroid by the patient or doctor. Signs of cancer within a nodule on ultrasound include "hypoechogenic" (solid) appearance, "taller than wide" size, microcalcifications (small bits of bright calcium), and irregular margins or borders. Fine needle aspiration has a high accuracy level for the diagnosis of cancer, approaching 95% in some studies. While there are multiple types of thyroid cancer, the most common types are papillary and follicular, both of which are called well differentiated thyroid cancers. Hurthle cell carcinoma is less common as is the medullary type, the latter being associated with a syndrome called multiple endocrine neoplasia 2. The most aggressive but fortunately uncommon type of thyroid cancer is called anaplastic. As opposed to patients with other types of thyroid cancer, most patients with anaplastic thyroid cancer have a small chance of surviving even one year following diagnosis. The remainder of the chapter will focus mainly on the most common types, papillary and follicular.

Staging

The AJCC TNM system is used for staging thyroid cancer. Initial management of patients should generally include laboratory measurements for general thyroid function with T3, T4, TSH, and sometimes blood levels of thyroglobulin. Other tests may include blood levels of calcium and, for patients with medullary thyroid cancer, calcitonin. An ultrasound of the neck is generally performed as initial imaging. Neck CT is sometimes obtained to evaluate regional anatomy including lymph nodes.

Unlike the staging of many other cancer disease sites, thyroid cancer staging includes age. In general, patients who are less than 45 years old fare much better than older patients. In fact, all patients younger than 45 are considered to have stage I disease unless they have metastasis (distant spread) which is considered stage II. At the other end of the spectrum, all patients with the anaplastic type of thyroid cancer are considered to have stage IV disease because of their near universally dismal outcomes with current treatment regimens.

In addition to young age, female sex, and complete surgical removal (which is common) predict a better outcome. While a few different prognostic systems have been used, one which has been widely utilized for years is known as AMES. The AMES risk criteria include age, metastasis, extent, and size. Based on these four criteria, patients may be grouped into low- and high-risk groups that have been shown to be predictive of survival. Long-term survival rates between low- and high-risk groups ranged from 98% down to 47% in one major center's 50-year experience that included over 1,000 patients.

Treatment

Surgical removal of the thyroid gland, total thyroidectomy, or near total removal is the initial treatment for most patients with cancer of this gland. Low-risk patients with early stage disease generally do well with surgery alone. High-risk patients may also undergo surgical removal of nearby lymph nodes on both sides of the neck if they are grossly enlarged or biopsy proven to contain cancer. Very small, single tumors may be treated with lobectomy, removal of a portion of the gland. An RCT from Italy revealed that patients who underwent video-assisted lobectomy had higher satisfaction, less post-operative pain, and shorter hospital stays than patients who were randomized to conventional lobectomy. In addition to the common surgical side effects, bleeding and infection, risks specific to thyroidectomy include changes in pitch and strength of voice, as well as a small chance of permanent hoarseness, due to injury of nearby nerves. There's also a risk of decreased parathyroid gland function called hypoparathyroidism, which necessitates patients taking calcium and vitamin D pills postoperatively.

Postoperatively, in patients deemed at high risk for return of their cancer, a radioactive iodine (RAI) ablation may then be performed. Treatment with RAI is recommended if the scan shows residual disease after surgery, or if the blood level of thyroglobulin remains high (more than 1 ng/ml). After treatment with RAI, another scan is done to ensure no residual disease. Repeat treatments may be given if there's evidence of residual thyroid on ultrasound or elevated thyroglobulin persists. For patients with iodine negative tumors, PET/CT scans have been found to be quite useful and may be predictive of survival.

External beam radiation therapy (RT) is used much less commonly for the treatment of thyroid cancer. It may be recommended as part of postoperative management for patients with multiple positive nodes, ECE, or positive surgical margins. External beam RT is also offered to patients with anaplastic thyroid cancer for palliation. Chemotherapy has not been found to be very effective for the treatment of most patients with thyroid cancer.

Peggy's Treatment and Outcome

Peggy was referred to a surgeon who specialized in the treatment of thyroid and other endocrine (glandular) cancers. He performed a total thyroidectomy and lymph node dissection, which confirmed cancer in the right lobe as well as two of 30 lymph nodes. She underwent radioactive iodine treatment postoperatively, which she tolerated well. Peggy is alive and well 16 years later. She continues to enjoy her part-time work as a special event planner.

UTERINE CANCER

Bonnie's Story

Bonnie was a 72-year-old homemaker who enjoyed baking and spending time with her many nieces and nephews. She had a history of high blood pressure, diabetes, and obesity. She had gone through menopause ("the change of life," as she described it) at age 55. However, over the past three months, she had noticed that she was getting vaginal bleeding again. She thought that was odd, since she hadn't had any periods for over 15 years. Bonnie went to her gynecologist, who performed a general pelvic examination that was unremarkable. Since the vaginal bleeding was clearly abnormal, she performed a biopsy of Bonnie's endometrium (inner lining of the uterus) which revealed adenocarcinoma, uterine cancer. (To be continued....)

Cancer of the uterus is one of the most common gynecologic malignancies. It's estimated to be diagnosed in 43,000 women in 2010 in the United States, with 8,000 deaths. The median age at diagnosis is 62 years old, and it's rarely diagnosed before age 30. A woman's lifetime risk of a uterine cancer diagnosis is 2.5%, or one in 40 women. The overall survival at five years from diagnosis for all stages combined is 83%, according to NCI's SEER statistics. This relatively high survival rate for uterine cancer is because over two-thirds of patients are diagnosed with localized disease and that group has a five-year survival rate of 96%. Five-year survival for those with regional spread is 67% and for those with metastatic uterine cancer is 17%.

Risks and Causes

Women who have early menarche (start of menstruation; "periods") and those who've never been pregnant and delivered a child (nulliparous) are at increased risk of developing uterine cancer. Women who have taken estrogen pills over years are also at increased risk, although this risk can be minimized by taking progestins for 10 or more days per month. Obesity is also closely linked to an increased risk of uterine cancer. Women who have polycystic ovary syndrome are at increased risk. Lastly, there's an approximately one in 200 chance of uterine cancer developing in patients who are taking a medication called tamoxifen to reduce their risk of breast cancer. In general, however, the large benefit of tamoxifen in decreasing future breast cancer risk greatly outweighs the small risk of developing uterine cancer for these women.

Signs and Symptoms

The most common symptom of cancer of the uterus is postmenopausal bleeding from the vagina. Once women have gone through menopause (the "change of life"), their menstruation ("periods") should stop altogether. Although there are occasionally benign reasons for postmenopausal vaginal bleeding, this symptom should always prompt a visit to the gynecologist.

Diagnosis

If a woman presents to her gynecologist with the complaint of postmenopausal bleeding, after the doctor does a thorough physical examination, an endometrial biopsy is usually performed. Contrary to what many people believe, a Pap test (which is done to screen for cancer of the cervix) is not a good test for uterine cancer. The gynecologist must directly biopsy the endometrium (inner lining of the uterus) in order to make a diagnosis of uterine cancer. Among the women who are diagnosed with uterine cancer, about 75% are found to have a type called endometrioid adenocarcinoma. Less commonly, patients may develop sarcomas of the uterus. The most common subtype of uterine sarcoma is called a carcinosarcoma or mixed muellerian tumor, while other types include leiomyosarcoma and stromal sarcoma.

Staging

Laboratory evaluation should include a complete blood count, serum chemistries including kidney and liver function, as well as a CA125 level. This blood test serves as a reasonable measure of the extent of microscopic uterine cancer that exists throughout the body and may be elevated in 60% of patients. If a woman's CA125 level is well above normal before surgery, there's a very good chance that cancer has spread outside the uterus. Imaging generally includes CT of the chest, abdomen and pelvis for patients with locally advanced disease, or if the primary tumor is a type of sarcoma. Patients also undergo cystoscopy and proctoscopy by a gynecologic oncologist, a surgical specialist in the treatment of female cancers. These tests involve direct visualization of the lining of the bladder and rectum, respectively, to ensure that cancer hasn't grossly invaded these nearby organs, which would indicate more advanced stage. While uterine cancer staging has classically been the FIGO system, the AJCC TNM system is now also widely used. Although most women have stage I disease that's limited to the endometrium or myometrium (deep muscle wall of the uterus), some patients present with more advanced diseased that's spread to other parts of the pelvis including lymph nodes. When metastases occur, they do so most commonly to the lungs or liver. The five-year survival by stage is approximately as follows: stage I-90%, stage II-70%, stage III-40%, and stage IV-10%.

After the stage, the next most important factor for predicting survival of uterine cancer is the grade of the tumor. Grade describes how aggressive the cells appear under the microscope, or how different the cells appear from normal uterine cells. Other factors that may predict prognosis for women with uterine cancer include patient age and overall condition, the presence or absence of cancer cells in lymphatic and blood vessel spaces, and the level of the patient's hemoglobin (the protein in blood that carries oxygen).

Treatment

The mainstay of treatment for cancer of the endometrium or uterus is surgical removal of the uterus, fallopian tubes, and ovaries by a gynecologic oncologist. This procedure is called a total abdominal hysterectomy, bilateral salpingo-oophorectomy, (TAH/BSO). During the surgery, sterile water is rinsed through the pelvis and abdomen, and the "washings" are sent with the surgical specimen so that the pathologist may review both to ensure that no cancer cells have escaped into these areas. Pelvic lymphadenectomy (removal or dissection of lymph nodes in the pelvis) has been part of the standard operation in the United States. At least two major RCTs have shown no benefit to pelvic lymphadenectomy in terms of survival or cancer recurrence. However, results of the lymph node dissection are often used in the United States to guide postoperative treatment recommendations. Comparisons of laparotomy (conventional open surgery) versus laparoscopy (making small incisions and placing a fiberoptic camera within the abdomen to guide surgery) have shown a small benefit to patients' quality of life with laparoscopy. Gynecologic oncologists at major cancer centers are now often performing these surgeries with robot assistance. In addition to the common surgical risks of bleeding, infection, and postoperative pain, side effects of hysterectomy for uterine cancer include nausea, small risk of bowel obstruction, and sexual dysfunction.

Very early stage patients don't require any postoperative treatment. Those with stage I disease that either invades deeply into the uterine muscle wall or has more aggressive, higher grade cancer cells may benefit from local postoperative internal radiation therapy (RT). These treatments are delivered to the top of the vagina, which is the most likely place for cancer to return following surgery. This type of internal RT is most commonly delivered on an outpatient basis by a radiation oncologist, a physician who specializes in the treatment of cancers with radiation. High dose rate (HDR) brachytherapy treatments are delivered in a few (usually three) outpatient weekly sessions. "Brachy" is Greek for "short," which describes the distance over which the internal RT travels. The treatment is called vaginal brachytherapy (VBT). The radiation oncologist places a cylinder into the patient's vagina which contains a central channel through which the radiation source travels from the HDR brachytherapy machine. The prescribed amount of RT is then delivered to the top portion of the vagina painlessly over a short time (five to 15 minutes) during each session. The RT dose to normal tissues even a couple of inches away from the top of the vagina with VBT is very low. Most women tolerate this treatment without acute side effects other than the mild discomfort of having the cylinder inserted into the vagina. An uncommon, long-term side effect called vaginal stenosis (scarring of the tissues at the top of the vagina) may cause pain. The risk of vaginal stenosis can be minimized by use of a vaginal dilator that keeps the tissues flexible and healthy.

Patients who have evidence of cancer cells outside the uterus but within the pelvis may benefit from postoperative pelvic external beam RT. As mentioned above, a pelvic lymphadenectomy is routinely performed during surgery in the United States in order to help guide recommendations for postoperative treatment. Most women who have aggressive features of the primary cancer but don't undergo a lymph node dissection should have postoperative RT to the pelvis in order to improve local control. In these patients, RT decreases the risk of cancer returning in the pelvis. Many women in Europe are treated in this manner, since pelvic lymphadenectomy is performed much less frequently there. However, even after a formal lymph node dissection is performed, some patients may benefit from postoperative pelvic RT. These include women with multiple positive lymph nodes and other high-risk features including tumor invasion of blood vessels or lymphatics extensively. In an RCT that enrolled over 500 women with uterine cancer, women whose tumors invaded nearby blood vessels had three times the risk of dying of their cancer. This same trial showed that for patients with stage I cancer, only those whose cancers invaded into deep uterine muscle or were high grade benefited from RT to the pelvis.

Postoperative pelvic RT was tested in another major RCT called the POR-TEC (postoperative radiation therapy in endometrial cancer) study. In this European trial, women did not have pelvic lymph nodes removed. Postoperative RT to the pelvis decreased the chance of cancer returning in the pelvis, but didn't improve patients' overall survival. The more recent PORTEC-2 trial from the Netherlands randomized patients with "high-intermediate risk" stage I and IIa uterine cancer to three VBT treatments versus four-and-a-half weeks of daily external beam RT to the pelvis. VBT resulted in fewer bowel side effects and similar survival to pelvic RT. Therefore, the investigators recommended that VBT should be the standard postoperative treatment for this group of women. Side effects of pelvic RT include acute irritation of the bladder and bowels that usually gets better by two to three weeks after RT is completed. There's a small risk of long-term problems with urination or bowel movements chronically after postoperative pelvic RT. The chance of a severe complication (such as one that would require surgery to repair) with standard pelvic RT is about 3%, according to the PORTEC trial results.

Patients who have advanced disease and are in good overall condition should receive postoperative chemotherapy for improved survival. Some of the medications that are used in the systemic treatment of uterine cancer include carboplatin, cisplatin, cyclophosphamide, doxorubicin, and paclitaxel. A very effective combination that's used in the United States is cisplatin and doxorubicin. A recent RCT performed by the Gynecologic Oncology Group (GOG) revealed no clear survival benefit to adding paclitaxel to the other two drugs. Another interesting GOG trial revealed that cisplatin and doxorubicin chemotherapy improved survival over RT to the whole abdomen for women with advanced disease. The combination of carboplatin and paclitaxel is also commonly used. Acute side effects of chemotherapy for uterine cancer include fatigue, nausea, vomiting, poor appetite, decreased blood counts, joint aches, and rare chance of long-term injury to heart, nerves, kidneys, or hearing.

Women who are diagnosed with metastatic uterine cancer that's spread to other organs, such as the liver or lungs, don't live any longer by having their uterus removed. Women with metastatic disease who are in good condition or are having symptoms are usually treated with similar chemotherapy agents to those with locally advanced disease. Side effects are also similar.

Bonnie's Uterine Cancer Treatment & Outcome

Bonnie's gynecologist referred her to a gynecologic oncologist, who performed a total abdominal hysterectomy, bilateral oophorectomy (TAH/BSO), with pelvic washings and lymph node dissection. Her tumor invaded into the uterine muscle layer to a depth of 1.5 cm of a total thickness of 2.0 cm and was grade 2. She had no cancer in multiple lymph nodes. Her stage was T1cN0M0. She recovered over four weeks and was referred to a radiation oncologist. This specialist recommended postoperative VBT to the top of the vagina to decrease the risk of the cancer returning there. She underwent three of these weekly outpatient treatments in the radiation oncology clinic with mild discomfort but no major side effects. Bonnie is alive without evidence of disease eight years later. She continues to win the county pie baking contest every year!

REFERENCES AND RESOURCES

PART I

AVOID MAJOR MISTAKES

U.S. Department of Health and Human Services. Public Health Service, National Toxicology Program. Report on Carcinogens, Eleventh Edition. 2005. Available at: http://ntp.niehs.nih.gov/ntp/roc/toc11.html.

Sasco AJ, Secretan MB, Straif K. Tobacco smoking and cancer: a brief review of epidemiological evidence. Lung Cancer 2004;45:S3-9.

Giovino GA. The tobacco epidemic in the United States. Am J Prev Med 2007; 33:S318-26.

Castellsague X. Natural history and epidemiology of HPV infection and cervical cancer. Gynecol Oncol 2008;110:S4-7.

Sallie R, Di Bisceglie AM. Viral hepatitis and hepatocellular carcinoma. Gastroenterol Clin North Am 1994;23:567-79.

Schutte K, Bornschein J, Malfertheiner P. Hepatocellular carcinoma-epidemiological trends and risk factors. Dig Dis 2009;27:80-92.

Engels EA, Pfeiffer RM, Goedert JJ, et al. Trends in cancer risk among people with AIDS in the United States 1980-2002. AIDS 2006;20:1645-54.

Seaberg EC, Wiley D, Martinez-Maza O, et al. Cancer incidence in the multicenter AIDS cohort study before and during the HAART era: 1984 to 2007. Cancer 2010 [Epub ahead of print]

Cader FZ, Kearns P, Young L, et al. The contribution of the Epstien-Barr virus to the pathogenesis of childhood lymphomas. Cancer Treat Rev 2010;36:348-53.

Samet JM. Radon and lung cancer. J Natl Cancer Inst 1989;81:745-57.

Lubin JH, Boice JD, Edling C, et al. Lung cancer in radon-exposed miners and estimation of risk from indoor exposure. J Natl Cancer Inst 1995;87:817-27.

Samet JM, Avila-Tang E, Boffetta P, et al. Lung cancer in never smokers: clinical epidemiology and environmental risk factors. Clin Cancer Res 2009;15:5626-45.

FUEL UP YOUR DEFENSE
NUTRITION & BREAST CANCER PREVENTION

Howe GR, Friedenreich CM, Jain M, Miller AB. A cohort study of fat intake and risk of breast cancer. J Natl Cancer Inst 1991;83:336-40.

Willett WC, Hunter DJ. Prospective studies of diet and breast cancer. Cancer 1994;74:1085-9.

Hunter DJ, Willett WC. Nutrition and breast cancer. Cancer Causes Control 1996;7:56-68.

Lee MM, Chang IY, Horng CF, et al. Breast cancer and dietary factors in Taiwanese women. Cancer Causes Control 2005;16:929-37.

Caan BJ, Aragaki A, Thomson CA, et al. Vasomotor symptoms, adoption of a low-fat dietary pattern, and risk of invasive breast cancer: a secondary analysis of the Women's Health Initiative randomized controlled dietary modification trial. J Clin Oncol 2009;27:4500-7.

Prentice RL, Caan B, Chlebowski et al. Low-fat dietary pattern and risk of invasive breast cancer: the Women's Health Initiative Randomized Controlled Dietary Modification Trial. JAMA 2006;295:629-42.

Smith-Warner SA, Spiegelman D, Yaun SS, et al. Intake of fruits and vegetables and risk of breast cancer: a pooled analysis of cohort studies. JAMA 2001;285:769-76.

Van Gils CH, Peeters PH, Bueno-de-Mesquita HB, et al. Consumption of vegetables and fruits and risk of breast cancer. JAMA 2005;293:183-93.

Mignone LI, Giovannucci E, Newcomb PA, et al. Dietary carotenoids and the risk of invasive breast cancer. Int J Cancer 2009;124:2929-37.

Nagel G, Linseisen J, van Gils CH, et al. Dietary beta-carotene, vitamin C and E intake and breast cancer risk in the European Prospective Investigation into Cancer and Nutrition (EPIC). Breast Cancer Res Treat 2010;119:753-65.

Bosetti C, Spertini L, Parpinei M, et al. Flavonoids and breast cancer risk in Italy. Cancer Epidemiol Biomarkers Prev 2005;14:805-8.

Dietary isoflavone intake and breast cancer risk in case-control studies in Japanese, Japanese Brazilians, and non-Japanese Brazilians. Breast Cancer Res Treat 2009;116:401-11.

Robien K, Cutler GJ, Lazovich D. Vitamin D intake and breast cancer risk in postmenopausal women: the Iowa Women's Health Study. Cancer Causes Control 2007;18:775-82.

Kesse-Guyot E, Bertrais S, Duperray B, et al. Dairy products, calcium, and the risk of breast cancer: results of the French SU.VI.MAX prospective study. Ann Nutr Metab 2007;51:139-45.

Nishio K, Niwa Y, Toyoshima H, et al. Consumption of soy foods and the risk of breast cancer: findings from the Japan Collaborative Cohort (JACC) Study. Cancer Cases Control 2007;18:801-8.

World Cancer Research Fund / American Institute for Cancer Research.

Food, Nutrition, Physical Activity, and the Prevention of Cancer: a Global Perspective. Washington DC: AICR, 2007

NUTRITION & GI (INCLUDING HEAD & NECK) CANCER PREVENTION

Negri E, Francheschi S, Bosetti C, et al. Selected micronutrients and oral and pharyngeal cancer. Int J Cancer 2000;86:122-7.

Pavia M, Pileggi C, Nobile CG, Angelillo IF. Association between fruit and vegetable consumption and oral cancer: a meta-analysis of observational studies. Am J Clin Nutr 2006;83:1126-34.

Pelucchi C, Talamini R, Levi F, et al. Fiber intake and laryngeal cancer risk. Ann Oncol 2003;14:162-7.

Garavello W, Lucenteforte E, Bosetti C, et al. Diet diversity and the risk of laryngeal cancer: a case-control study from Italy and Switzerland. Oral Oncol 2009;45:85-9.

Chen YK, Lee CH, Wu IC, et al. Food intake and the occurrence of squamous cell carcinoma in different sections of esophagus in Taiwanese men. Nutrition 2009; 25:753-61.

De Stafani E, Deneo-Pellegrini H, Ronco AL, et al. Food groups and risk of squamous cell carcinoma of the oesophagus: a case-control study in Uruguay. Br J Cancer 2003;89:1209-14.

Castellsague X, Munoz N, De Stefani E, et al. Influence of mate drinking, hot beverages and diet on esophageal cancer risk in South America. Int J Cancer 2000;88:658-64.

Gonzalez CA, Jakszyn P, Pera G, et al. Meat intake and risk of stomach and esophageal adenocarcinoma within the European Prospective Investigation Into Cancer and Nutrition (EPIC). J Natl Cancer Inst 2006;98:345-54.

Gonzalez CA, Pera G, Agudo A, et al. Fruit and vegetable intake and the risk of stomach and oesophageal adenocarcinoma in the European Prospective Investigation into Cancer and Nutrition (EPIC-EURGAST). Int J Cancer 2006;118:2559-66.

Buckland G, Agudo A, Lujan L, et al. Adherence to a Mediterranean diet and risk of gastric adenocarcinoma within the European Prospective Investigation into Cancer and Nutrition (EPIC) cohort study. Am J Clin Nutr 2010;91:381-390.

Nouraie M, Pitinen P, Kamangar F, et al. Fruits, vegetables, and antioxidants and risk of gastric cancer among male smokers. Cancer Epidemiol Biomarkers Prev 2005;14:2087-92.

Navarro Silvera SA, Mayne ST, Risch H, et al. Food group intake and risk of subtypes of esophageal and gastric cancer. Int J Cancer 2008;123:852-60.

Lunet N, Valbuena C, Vieira AL, et al. Fruit and vegetable consumption and gastric cancer by location and histological type: case-control and meta-analysis. Eur J Cancer 2007;16:312-27.

Nishimoto IN, Hamada GS, Kowalski LP, et al. Risk factors for stomach cancer in Brazil (I): a case-control study among non-Japanese Brazilians in Sao Paulo. Jpn J Clin Oncol 2002;32:277-83.

Hamada GS, Kowalski LP, Nishimoto IN, et al. Risk factors for stomach cancer in Brazil (II): a case-control study among Japanese Brazilians in Sao Paulo. Jpn J Clin Oncol 2002;32:284-90.

Blot WJ, Li JY, Taylor PR, et al. Nutrition intervention trials in Linxian, China: supplementation with specific vitamin/mineral combinations, cancer incidence, and disease-specific mortality in the general population. J Natl Cancer Inst 1993;85:1483-92.

Taylor PR, Li B, Dawsey SM, et al. Prevention of esophageal cancer: the nutrition intervention trials in Linxian, China, Linxian Nutrition Intervention Trials Study Group. Cancer Res 1994;54:2029s-2031s.

Mayne ST, Risch HA, Dubrow R, et al. Carbonated soft drink consumption and risk of esophageal adenocarcinoma. J Natl Cancer Inst 2006;98:72-5.

Wu AH, Yang D, Pike MC. A meta-analysis of soyfoods and risk of stomach cancer: the problem of potential cofounders. Cancer Epidemiol Biomarkers Prev 2000;9:1054-8.

Norat T, Bingham S, Ferrari P, et al. Meat, fish, and colorectal cancer risk: the European Prospective Investigation into cancer and nutrition. J Natl Cancer Inst 2005;97:906-16.

Gonzalez CA. the European Prospective Investigation into Cancer and Nutrition (EPIC). Public Health Nutr 2006;9:124-6.

Cross AJ, Leitzmann MF, Gail MH, et al. A prospective study of red and processed meat in relation to cancer risk. PLoS Med 2007;4:e325.

Sandhu MS, White IR, McPherson K. Systematic review of the prospective cohort studies and meat consumption and colorectal cancer risk: a meta-analytical approach. Cancer Epidemiol Biomarkers Prev 2001;10:439-46.

Francheschi S, Favero A, La Vecchia C, et al. Food groups and risk of colorectal cancer in Italy. Int J Cancer 1997;72:56-61.

Braga C, La Vecchia C, Francheschi S, et al. Olive oil, other seasoning fats, and the risk of colorectal carcinoma. Cancer 1998;82:448-53.

Koushik A, Hunter DJ, Spiegelman D, et al. Fruits, vegetables, and colon cancer risk in a pooled analysis of 14 cohort studies. J Natl Cancer Inst 2007;99:1471-83.

Hara M, Hanaoka T, Kobayashi M, et al. Cruciferous vegetables, mushrooms, and gastrointestinal cancer risks in a multicenter, hospital-based case-control study in Japan. Nutr Cancer 2003;46:138-47.

Beresford SA, Johnson KC, Ritenbaugh C, et al. Low-fat dietary pattern and risk of colorectal cancer: the Women's Health Initiative Randomized Controlled Dietary Modification Trial. JAMA 2006;295:643-54.

Prentice RL, Thomson CA< Caan B, et al. Low-fat dietary pattern and cancer incidence in the Women's Health Initiative Dietary Modification Randomized Controlled Trial. J Natl Cancer Inst 2007;99:1534-43.

NUTRITION & OVARIAN & UTERINE CANCER PREVENTION

Pan SY, Ugnat AM, Mao Y, et al. A case-control study of diet and the risk of ovarian cancer. Cancer Epidemiol Biomarkers Prev 2004;13:1521-7.

Bosetti C, Negri E, Francheschi S, et al. Diet and ovarian cancer risk: a case-control study in Italy. Int J Cancer 2001;93:911-5.

Schulz M, Lahmann PH, Boeing H, et al. Fruit and vegetable consumption and risk of epithelial ovarian cancer: the European Prospective Investigation into Cancer and Nutrition. Cancer Epidemiol Biomarkers Prev 2005;14:2531-5.

Gates MA, Tworoger SS, Hecht JL, et al. A prospective study of dietary flavonoid intake and incidence of epithelial ovarian cancer. Int J Cancer 2007;121:2225-32.

Rossi M, Negri E, Lagiou P, et al. Flavonoids and ovarian cancer risk: a case-control study in Italy. Int J Cancer 2008;123:895-8.

Huncharek M, Klassen H, Kupelnick B. Dietary beta-carotene intake and the risk of epithelial ovarian cancer: a meta-analysis of 3,782 subjects from five observational studies. In Vivo 2001'15:339-43.

Levi F, Francheschi S, Negri E, La Vecchia C. Dietary factors and the risk of endometrial cancer. Cancer 1993;71:3575-81.

Lucenteforte E, Talamini R, Montella M, et al. Macronutrients, fatty acids, and cholesterol intake and endometrial cancer. Ann Oncol 2008;19:168-72.

McCullough ML, Bandera EV, Moore DF, Kushi LH. Vitamin D and calcium intake in relation to risk of endometrial cancer: a systematic review of the literature.

NUTRITION & LUNG CANCER PREVENTION

Miller AB, Altenburg HP, Bueno-de-Mesquita B, et al. Fruits and vegetables and lung cancer: Findings from the European Prospective Investigation into Cancer and Nutrition. Int J Cancer 2004;108:269-76.

Brennan P, Fortes C, Butler J, et al. A multicenter case-control study of diet and lung cancer among non-smokers. Cancer Causes Control 2000;11:49-58.

Neuhouser ML, Patterson RE, Thornquist MD, et al. Fruits and vegetables are associated with lower lung cancer risk only in the placebo arm of the beta-carotene and retinol efficacy trial (CARET). Cancer Epidemiol Biomarkers Prev 2003;12:350-8.

Gallicchio L, Boyd K, Matanowski G, et al. Carotenoids and the risk of developing lung cancer: a systematic review. Am J Clin Nutr 2008;88:372-83.

Reid ME, Duffield-Lillico AJ, Garland L, et al. Selenium supplementation and lung cancer incidence: an update of the nutritional prevention of cancer trial. Cancer Epidemiol Biomarkers Prev 2002;11:1285-91.

Wright ME, Mayne ST, Stolzenberg-Solomon RZ, et al. Development of a comprehensive dietary antioxidant index and application to lung cancer in a cohort of male smokers. Am J Epidemiol 2004;160:66-78.

Kamangar F, Qiao YL, Yu B, et al. Lung cancer chemoprevention: a randomized, double-blind trial in Linxian, China. Cancer Epidemiol Biomarkers Prev 2006;15:1562-4.

Rohrmann S, Linseisen J, Boshuizen HC, et al. Ethanol intake and risk of lung cancer in the European Prospective Investigation into Cancer and Nutrition (EPIC). Am J Epidemiol 2006;164:1103-14.

NUTRITION & PROSTATE CANCER PREVENTION

Allen NE, Key TJ, Appleby PN, et al. Animal foods, protein, calcium and prostate cancer risk: the European Prospective Investigation into Cancer and Nutrition. Br J Cancer 2008;98:1574-81.

Kesse E, Bertrias S, Astorg P, et al. Dairy products, calcium and phosphorus intake, and the risk of prostate cancer: results of the French prospective SU.VI.MAX (Supplementation en Vitamines et Mineraux Antioxydants) study. Br J Nutr 2006; 95:539-45.

Tzonou A, Signorello LB, Lagiou P, et al. Diet and cancer of the prostate: a case-control study in Greece. Int J Cancer 1999;80:704-8.

Chan JM, Pietinen P, Virtanen M, et al. Diet and prostate cancer risk in a cohort of smokers, with a specific focus in calcium and phosphorus (Finland). Cancer Causes Control 2000;11:859-67.

Ahn J, Albenes D, Peters U, et al. Dairy products, calcium intake, and risk of prostate cancer in the prostate, lung, colorectal, and ovarian cancer screening trial. Cancer Epidemiol Biomarkers Prev 2007;16:2623-30.

Jain MG, Hislop GT, Howe GR, Ghadirian P. Plant foods, antioxidants, and prostate cancer risk: findings from case-control studies in Canada. Nutr Cancer 1999;34:173-84.

Ambrosini GL de Klerk NH, Fritschi L, et al. Fruit, vegetable, vitamin A intakes, and prostate cancer risk. Prostate Cancer Prostatic Dis 2008;11:61-6.

Cross AJ, Peters U, Kirsh VA, et al. A prospective study of meat and meat mutagens and prostate cancer risk. Cancer Res 2005;15:1179-84.

Kirsh VA, Mayne ST, Peters U, et al. A prospective study of lycopene and tomato product intake and risk of prostate cancer. Cancer Epidemiol Biomarkers Prev 2006;15:92-8.

Rohrmann S, Linseisen J, Key TJ, et al. Alcohol consumption and the risk of prostate cancer in the European Prospective Investigation into Cancer and Nutrition. Cancer Epidemiol Biomarkers Prev 2008;17:1282-7.

Suzuki R, Allen NE, Key TJ, et al. A prospective analysis of the association between dietary fiber intake and prostate cancer risk in EPIC. Int J Cancer 2009;124:245-9.

Weinstein SJ, Wright ME, Lawson KA, et al. Serum and dietary vitamin E in relation to prostate cancer risk. Cancer Epidemiol Biomarkers Prev 2007;16:1253-9.

Lawson KA, Wright ME, Subar A, et al. Multivitamin use and risk of prostate cancer in the National Institutes of Health-AARP Diet and Health Study. J Natl Cancer Inst 2007;99:754-64.

Clark LC, Dalkin B, Krongrad A, et al. Decreased incidence of prostate cancer with selenium supplementation: results of a double blind cancer prevention trial. Br J Urol 1998;81:730-4.

Moyad MA. Selenium and vitamin E supplementation for prostate cancer: evidence or embellishment. Urology 2002;59:9-19.

World Cancer Research Fund / American Institute for Cancer Research.

Food, Nutrition, Physical Activity, and the Prevention of Cancer: a Global Perspective. Washington DC: AICR, 2007

TAKE THE BALL BY THE HORNS

Rockhill B, Willett WC, Hunter DJ, et al. A prospective study of recreational physical activity and breast cancer risk. Arch Intern Med 1999;159:2290-6.

Peplonske B, Lissowska J, Hartmen TJ, et al. Adulthood lifetime physical activity and breast cancer. Epidemiology 2008;19:226-36.

Thune I, Furberg AS. Physical activity and cancer risk: dose-response and cancer, all sites and site-specific. Med Sci Sports Exerc. 2001;33:S530-50.

Friedenreich Cm, Cust AE. Physical activity and breast cancer risk: impact of timing, type, and dose of activity and population subgroup effects. Br J Sports Med 2008; 42:636-47.

Bernstein L, Patel AV, Ursin G, et al. Lifetime recreational exercise activity and breast cancer risk among black women and white women. J Natl Cancer Inst 2005;97:1671-9.

Key T, Appleby P, Barnes I, et al. Endogenous sex hormones and breast cancer in postmenopausal women: reanalysis of nine prospective studies. J Natl Cancer Inst 2002;94:606.

McTiernan A, Tworoger SS, Ulrich CM, et al. Effect of exercise on serum estrogens in postmenopausal women: a 12-minth randomized clinical trial. Cancer Res 2004; 64:2923-8.

Friedenreich CM, Woolcott CG, McTiernan A, et al. Alberta physical activity and breast cancer prevention trial: sex hormone changes in a year-long exercise intervention among postmenopausal women. J Clin Oncol 2010;28:1458-66.

Platz EA, Willett WC, Colditz GA, et al. Proportion of colon cancer risk that might be preventable in a cohort of middle-aged US men. Cancer Causes Control 2000;11:579-88.

Chan AT, Giovannucci EL. Primary prevention of colorectal cancer. Gastroenterology 2010;138:2029-43.

Huxley RR, Ansary-Moghaddam A, Clifton P, et al. The impact of dietary and life-style risk factors on the risk of colorectal cancer: a quantitative overview of the epidemiological evidence. Int J Cancer 2009;125:171-80.

Thune I, Lund E. Physical activity and risk of colorectal cancer in men and women. Br J Cancer 1996;73:1134-40.

Colbert LH, Hartman TJ, Malila N, et al. Physical activity in relation to cancer of the colon and rectum in a cohort of male smokers. Cancer Epidemiol Biomarkers Prev 2001;10:265-8.

Martinez ME, Giovannucci E, Spiegelman D, et al. Leisure-time physical activity, body size, and colon cancer in women. Nurses' health Study Research Group. J Natl Cancer Inst 1997;89:948-55.

Lee IM, Sesso HD, Paffenbarger RS. Physical activity and risk of lung cancer. Int J Epidemiol 1999;28:620-5.

Colbert LH, Martman TJ, Tangrea JA, et al. Physical activity and lung cancer risk in male smokers. Int J Cancer 2002;98:770-3.

Tardon A, Lee WJ, Delgado-Rodriguez M, et al. Leisure-time physical activity and lung cancer: a meta-analysis. Cancer Causes Control 2005;16:398-97.

Hartman TJ, Albanes D, Rautalahti M, et al. Physical activity and prostate cancer in the Alpha-Tocopherol, Beta-Carotne (ATBC) Cancer Prevention Study (Finland). Cancer Causes Control 1998;9:11-18.

Johnson NF, Tjonneland A, Thomsen BL, et al. Physical activity and risk of prostate cancer in the European Prospective Investigation into Cancer and Nutrition (EPIC) cohort. Int J Cancer 2009;125:902-8.

Jian L, Shen ZJ, Lee AH, Binns CW. Moderate physical activity and prostate cancer risk: a case-control study in China. Eur J Epidemiol 2005;20:155-60.

Pierotti B, Altieri A, Talamini R, et al. Lifetime physical activity and prostate cancer risk. Int J Cancer 2005;114:639-42.

Giovannucci E, Leitzmann M, Spiegelman D, et al. A prospective study of physical activity and prostate cancer in male health professionals. Cancer Res 1998; 58:5117-22.

Liu S, Lee IM, Linson P, et al. A prospective study of physical activity and risk of prostate cancer in US physicians. Int J Epidemiol 2000;29:29-35.

Oliveria SA, Lee IM. Is exercise beneficial in the prevention of prostate cancer? Sports Med 1997;23:271-8.

Friedenreich CM, Thune I. A review of physical activity and prostate cancer risk. Cancer Causes Control 2001;12:461-75.

Torti DC, Matheson GO. Exercise and prostate cancer. Sports med 2004;34:363-9.

THE NEXT BEST THING

American Medical Association Council on Scientific Affairs. *Commercialized Medical Screening (Report A-03)*. Available at: http://www.ama-assn.org/ama/pub/category/13628.html.

Smith RA, Cokkinides V, Brooks D, et al. Cancer screening in the United States, 2010: a review of current American Cancer Society guidelines, and issues in cancer screening. CA Cancer J Clin 2010;60:99-119.

MAMMOGRAPHY

Miller AB. Is routine mammography screening appropriate for women 40-49 years of age? Am J Prev Med 1991;7:55-62.

Elmore JG, Armstrong K, Lehman CD, Fletcher SW. Screening for breast cancer. JAMA 2005;293:1245-1256.

Mushlin AI, Kouides RW, Shapiro DE. Estimating the accuracy of screening mammography: a meta-analysis. Am J Prev Med 1998;14:143-153.

Gotzsche PC, Nielsen M. Screening for breast cancer with mammography. Cochrane Database Syst Rev 2009;CD001877.

Armstrong K, Moye E, Williams S, et al. Screening mammography in women 40 to 49 years of age: a systematic review for the American College of Physicians. Ann Intern Med 2007;146:516-526.

Miller AB, To T, Baines CJ, et al.: The Canadian National Breast Screening Study-1: breast cancer mortality after 11 to 16 years of follow-up. A randomized screening trial of mammography in women age 40 to 49 years. Ann Intern Med 2002;137:305-12.

Miller AB, Baines CJ, To T, et al.: Canadian National Breast Screening Study: 2. Breast cancer detection and death rates among women aged 50 to 59 years. CMAJ 1992;147: 1477-88.

Nystrom L, Andersson I, Bjurstam, et al. Long-term effects of mammography screening: updated overview of the Swedish randomized trials. Lancet 2002;359:909-919.

Moss SM, Cuckle H, Evans A, et al. Effect of mammographic screening from age 40 years on breast cancer mortality at 10 years' follow-up: a randomized controlled trial. Lancet 2006;368:2053-2060.

Joensuu H, Lehtimäki T, Holli K, et al.: Risk for distant recurrence of breast cancer detected by mammography screening or other methods. JAMA 2004;292:1064-73.

Shen Y, Yang Y, Inoue LY, et al.: Role of detection method in predicting breast cancer survival: analysis of randomized screening trials. J Natl Cancer Inst 97 2005;97:1195-1203.

Wishart GC, Greenberg DC, Britton PD, et al.: Screen-detected vs symptomatic breast cancer: is improved survival due to stage migration alone? Br J Cancer 2008;98:1741-4.

Esserman L, Kerlikowske K. Should we recommend screening mammography for women aged 40 to 49? Oncology 1996;10:357-364.

Nelson HD, Tyne K, Naik A, et al. Screening for breast cancer: an update for the U.S. Preventive Services Task Force. Ann Intern Med 2009;151:727-737.

U.S. Preventive Services Task Force. Screening for breast cancer: U.S. Preventive Services Task Force recommendation statement. Ann Intern Med 2009;151:716-726.

Smith RA, Cokkinides V, Brooks D, et al. Cancer screening in the United States, 2010: a review of current American Cancer Society guidelines, and issues in cancer screening. CA Cancer J Clin 2010;60:99-119.

Kalager M, Zelen M, Langmark F, Adami HO. Effect of screening mammography on breast-cancer mortality in Norway. N Eng J Med 2010;363:1203-10.

PSA

Wolf AM, Wender RC, Etzioni RB, et al. American Cancer Society guideline for the early detection of prostate cancer: update 2010. CA Cancer J Clin 2010;60:70-98.

Green KL, Albertsen PC, Babaian RJ, et al. Prostate specific antigen best practice statement: 2009 update. J Urol 2009;182:2232-2241.

Thompson IM, Pauler D, Goodman PJ et al., Prevalence of prostate cancer among men with a prostate-specific antigen level <4.0 ng per milliliter. N Eng J Med 2004;350:2239-2246.

Catalona WJ, Smith DS, Ratliff TL, et al. Measurement of prostate-specific antigen in serum as a screening test for prostate cancer. N Eng J Med. 1991;324:1156–1161.

Crawford ED, Pinsky PF, Chia D, et al. Prostate specific antigen changes as related to the initial prostate specific antigen: data from the prostate, lung, colorectal and ovarian cancer screening trial. J Urol. 2006;175:1286–1290.

Thompson IM, Ankerst DP, Chi C, et al. Assessing prostate cancer risk: results from the Prostate Cancer Prevention Trial. J Natl Cancer Inst. 2006;98:529–534.

Carter HB, Pearson JD, Metter EJ, et al. Longitudinal evaluation of prostate-specific antigen levels in men with and without prostate disease. JAMA 1992;267:2215–2220.

Carter HB, Ferrucci L, Kettermann A, et al. Detection of life-threatening prostate cancer with prostate-specific antigen velocity during a window of curability. J Natl Cancer Inst 2006;98:1521–1527.

Vickers AJ, Savage C, O'Brien MF, Lilja H. Systematic review of pretreatment prostate-specific antigen velocity and doubling time as predictors for prostate cancer. J Clin Oncol 2009;27:398–403.

Vickers A, Cronin A, Roobol M, et al. Reducing unnecessary biopsy during prostate cancer screening using a four-kallikrein panel: an independent replication. J Clin Oncol 2010;28:2493-2498.

Draisma G, Etzioni R, Tsodikov A, et al. Lead time and overdiagnosis in prostate-specific antigen screening: importance of methods and context. J Natl Cancer Inst 2009;101:374–383.

Lin K, Lipsitz R, Miller T, et al. Benefits and harms of prostate-specific antigen screening for prostate cancer: an evidence update for the U.S. Preventative Services Task Force. Ann Intern Med 2008;149:137.

Cooperburg MR, Broering JM, Kantoff PW, Carroll PR. Contemporary trends in low risk prostate cancer: risk assessment and treatment. J Urol 2007;178:S14-19.

Andriole GL, Crawford ED, Grubb RL et al. Mortality results from a randomized prostate-cancer screening trial. N Eng J Med 2009;360:1310-9.

Schröder FH, Hugosson J, Roobol MJ, et al. Screening and prostate-cancer mortality in a randomized European study. N Eng J Med 2009;360:1320-8.

Etzioni R, Feuer E. Studies of prostate-cancer mortality: caution advised. Lancet Oncol 2008;9:407–409.

Collin SM, Martin RM, Metcalfe C, et al. Prostate-cancer mortality in the USA and UK in 1975–2004: an ecological study. Lancet Oncol 2008;9:445–452.

Kerkhof M, Roobol MJ, Steyerberg EW, Cuzick J, Schroder FH. Secondary analysis of the European Randomised Study of Screening for Prostate Cancer (ERSPC)—effect of prostate cancer screening on the development of metastases after adjustment for non-compliance and contamination [abstract]. J Urol 2009;181:233. Abstract 648

Grubb RL 3rd, Pinsky PF, Greenlee RT, et al. Prostate cancer screening in the Prostate, Lung, Colorectal and Ovarian cancer screening trial: update on findings from the initial four rounds of screening in a randomized trial. BJU Int 2008;102:1524–1530

Hankey BF, Feuer EJ, Clegg LX, et al. Cancer surveillance series: interpreting trends in prostate cancer—part I: evidence of the effects of screening in recent prostate cancer incidence, mortality, and survival rates. J Natl Cancer Inst 1999;91:1017–1024.

PAP

Vilos GA. The history of the Papanicolaou smear and the odyssey of George and Andromache Papanicolaou. Obstet Gynecol 1998;91:479-483.

Koss LG. The Papanicolaou test for cervical cancer detection. A triumph and a tragedy. JAMA 1989;261:737-743.

Smith RA, Cokkinides V, Brooks D, et al. Cancer screening in the United States, 2010: a review of current American Cancer Society guidelines, and issues in cancer screening. CA Cancer J Clin 2010;60:99-119.

Siebers AG, Klinkhamer PJ, Grefte JM, et al. Comparison of liquid-based cytology with conventional cytology for detection of cervical cancer precursors: a randomized controlled trial. JAMA 2009;302:1757-1764.

Arbyn M, Bergeron C, Klinkhamer P, et al. Liquid compared with conventional cervical cytology: a systematic review and meta-analysis. Obstet Gynecol 2008;111:167-177.

Cum CP, Abbott DW, Quade BJ. Cervical cancer screening: from the Papanicolaou smear to the vaccine era. J Clin Oncol 2003;21:224s-230s.

Mayrand MH, Duarte-Fanco E, Rodrigues I, et al. Human papillomavirus DNA versus Papanicolaou screening tests for cervical cancer. N Eng J Med 2007; 357:1579-1588.

Naucler P, Ryd W, Tornberg S, et al. Human papillomavirus and Papanicolaou tests to screen for cervical cancer. N Eng J Med 2007;357:1589-1597.

Naucler P, Ryd W, Tornberg S, et al. Efficacy of HPV DNA testing with cytology triage and/or repeat HPV DNA testing in primary cervical cancer screening. J Natl Cancer Inst 2009;101:88-99.

COLONOSCOPY

Kronberg O, Fenger C, Olsen J, et al. Randomized study of screening for colorectal cancer with faecal-occult-blood test. Lancet 1996;348:1467-1471.

Hardcastle JD, Chamberlain JO, Robinson MH, et al. Randomized controlled trial of faecal-occult-blood screening for colorectal cancer. Lancet 1996;348:1472-1477.

Mandel JS, Bond JH, Church TR, et al. Reducing mortality from colorectal cancer by screening for fecal occult blood. Minnesota Colon Cancer Control Study. N Eng J Med 328:1365-1371.

Lieberman DA, Weiss DG. One-time screening for colorectal cancer with combined fecal occult-blood testing and examination of the distal colon. N Eng J Med 2001; 345:555-560.

Lieberman DA, Weiss DG, Bond JH, et al. Use of colonoscopy to screen asymptomatic adults for colorectal cancer. Veterans Affairs Cooperative Study Group 380. N Eng J Med 2000;343:162-168.

Imperiale TF, Wagner DR, Lin CY, et al. Risk of advanced proximal neoplasms in asymptomatic adults according to the distal colorectal findings. N Eng J Med 2000; 343:169-174.

Schoenfeld P, Cash B, Flood A, et al. Colonoscopic screening of average risk women for colorectal neoplasia. N Eng J Med 2005;352:2061-2068.

Frazier AL, Colditz GA, Fuchs CS, Kuntz KM. Cost-effectiveness of screening for colorectal cancer in the general population. JAMA 2000;84:1954-1961.

Sonnenberg A, Delco F, Inadomi JM. Cost-effectiveness of colonoscopy in screening for colorectal cancer. Ann Intern Med 2000;133:573-584.

PART II

BLADDER CANCER

Altekruse SF, Kosary CL, Krapcho M, Neyman N, Aminou R, Waldron W, Ruhl J, Howlader N, Tatalovich Z, Cho H, Mariotto A, Eisner MP, Lewis DR, Cronin K, Chen HS, Feuer EJ, Stinchcomb DG, Edwards BK (eds). SEER Cancer Statistics Review, 1975-2007, National Cancer Institute. Bethesda, MD, http://seer.cancer.gov/csr/1975_2007/, based on November 2009 SEER data submission, posted to the SEER web site, 2010

Silverman DT, Hartge P, Morrison AS, Devessa SS. Epidemiology of bladder cancer. Hematol Oncol Clin North Am 1992;6:1-30.

Urinary Bladder. In: Edge SB, Byrd DR, Compton CC, eds. *AJCC Cancer Staging Manual.* 7th ed. New York, NY: Springer, 2010, pp. 497-510.

Herr HW, Schwalb DM, Zhang ZF, et al. Intravesical bacillus Calmette-Guerin therapy prevents tumor progression and death from superficial bladder cancer: ten-year follow-up of a prospective randomized trial. J Clin Oncol 1995;13:1404-8.

Cheng CW, Chan SF, Chan LW, et al. Twelve-year follow up of a randomized prospective trial comparing bacillus Calmette-Guerin and epirubicin as adjuvant therapy in superficial bladder cancer. Int J Urol 2005;12:449-55.

Duchek M, Johansson R, Jahnson S, et al. Bacillus Calmette-Guerin is superior to a combination of epirubicin and interferon-alpha2b in the intravesical treatment of patients with stage T1 urinary bladder cancer. A prospective, randomized, Nordic study. Eur Urol 2010;57:25-31.

Steven K, Paulson AL. The orthotopic Koch ileal neobladder: functional results, urodynamic features, complications and survival in 166 men. J Urol 2000;164:288-95.

Kaufman DS, Shipley WU, Griffin PP, et al. Selective bladder preservation by combination treatment of invasive bladder cancer. N Eng J Med 1993;329:1377-82.

Shipley WU, Winter KA, Kaufman DS, et al. Phase III trial of neoadjuvant chemotherapy in patients with invasive bladder cancer treated with selective bladder preservation by combined radiation therapy and chemotherapy: initial results of Radiation Therapy Oncology Group 89-03. J Clin Oncol 1998;16:3576-83.

Efstathiou JA, Kyounghwa B, Shipley WU, et al. Late pelvic toxicity after bladder-sparing therapy in patients with invasive bladder cancer: RTOG 89-03, 95-06, 97-06, 99-06. J Clin Oncol 2009;27:4055-61.

Von der Masse H, Sengelov L, Roberts JT, et al. Long-term survival results of a randomized trial comparing gemcitabine plus cisplatin, with methotrexate, vinblastine, doxorubicin, plus cisplatin in patients with bladder cancer. J Clin Oncol 2005;23:4602-8.

BRAIN METASTASES AND PRIMARY BRAIN TUMORS

Altekruse SF, Kosary CL, Krapcho M, Neyman N, Aminou R, Waldron W, Ruhl J, Howlader N, Tatalovich Z, Cho H, Mariotto A, Eisner MP, Lewis DR, Cronin K, Chen HS, Feuer EJ, Stinchcomb DG, Edwards BK (eds). SEER Cancer Statistics Review, 1975-2007, National Cancer Institute. Bethesda, MD, http://seer.cancer.gov/csr/1975_2007/, based on November 2009 SEER data submission, posted to the SEER web site, 2010

Patchell RA, Tibbs PA, Walsh JW, et al. A randomized trial of surgery in the treatment of single metastases to the brain. New Eng J Med 1990;322:494-500.

Kondziolka D, Patel A, Lunsford LD, et al. Stereotactic radiosurgery plus whole brain radiotherapy versus radiotherapy alone for patients with multiple brain metastases. Int J Radiat Oncol Biol Phys 1999;45:427-34.

Andrews DW, Scott CB, Sperduto PW, et al. Whole brain radiation therapy with or without stereotactic radiosurgery boost for patients with one to three brain metastases: phase III results of the RTOG 9508 randomized trial. Lancet 2004;363:1665-72.

Patchell RA, Tibbs PA, Regine WF, et al. Postoperative radiotherapy in the treatment of single metastases to the brain: a randomized trial. JAMA 1998;280:1485-9.

Walker MD, Green SB, Byar DP, et al. Randomized comparisons of radiotherapy and nitrosoureas for the treatment of malignant glioma after surgery. N Eng J Med 1980;303:1323-9.

Stupp R, Mason WP, van den Bent MJ, et al. Radiotherapy plus concomitant and adjuvant temozolomide for glioblastoma. New Eng J Med 2005;352:987-96.

Stupp R, Hegi ME, Mason WP, et al. Effects of radiotherapy with concomitant and adjuvant temozolomide versus radiotherapy alone on survival in glioblastoma in randomized phase III study: 5-year analysis of the EORTC-NCIC trial. Lancet Oncol 2009; 10:459-66.

Karim AB, Maat B, Hatlevoll R, et al. A randomized trial on dose response in radiation therapy of low-grade cerebral glioma: European Organization for Research and Treatment of Cancer (EORTC) Study 22844. Int J Radiat Oncol Biol Phys 1996;36:549-56.

Karim AB, Afra D, Cornu P, et al. Randomized trial on the efficacy of radiotherapy for cerebral low-grade glioma in the adult: European Organization for Research and Treatment of Cancer (EORTC) Study BR04: an interim analysis. Int J Radiat Oncol Biol Phys 2002;52:316-324.

Shaw E, Arusell R, Scheithauser BW, et al. Prospective randomized trial of low-versus high-dose radiation therapy in adults with supratentorial low grade glioma: initial report of the North Central Cancer Treatment Group/Radiation Therapy Oncology Group/Eastern Cooperative Oncology Group study. J Clin Oncol 2002;20:2267-76.

Stafford SL, Perry A, Suman VJ, et al. Primarily resected meningiomas: outcome and prognostic factors in 581 Mayo Clinic patients, 1978 through 1988. Mayo Clin Proc 1998;73:936-42.

Goldsmith BJ, Wara WM, Wilson CB, Larson DA. Postoperative irradiation for subtotally resected meningiomas. A retrospective analysis of 140 patients treated from 1967 to 1990. J Neurosurg 1994;80:195-201.

Kondziolka D, Levy EI, Niranjan A, et al. Long-term outcomes after meningioma radiosurgery: physician and patient perspectives. J Neurosurg 1999;91:44-50.

Cook DM. Pituitary tumors: diagnosis and therapy. CA Cancer J Clin 1983;33:215-36.

Meijer OW, Vandertop WP, Baayen JC, Slotman BJ. Single-fraction vs. fraction-ated linac-based stereotactic radiosurgery for vestibular schwannoma: a single institution study. In t J Radiat Oncol Biol Phys 2003;56:1390-6.

Niranjan A, Mathieu D, Flickinger JC, et al. Hearing preservation after intracanalicu-lar vestibular schwannoma radiosurgery. Neurosurgery 2008;63:1054-62.

Combs SE, Weizel T, Schulz-Ertner D, et al. Differences in clinical results after LINAC-based single-dose radiosurgery versus fractionated stereotactic radiotherapy for patients with vestibular schwannomas. Int J Radiat Oncol Biol Phys 2010;76:193-200.

BREAST CANCER

Altekruse SF, Kosary CL, Krapcho M, Neyman N, Aminou R, Waldron W, Ruhl J, Howlader N, Tatalovich Z, Cho H, Mariotto A, Eisner MP, Lewis DR, Cronin K, Chen HS, Feuer EJ, Stinchcomb DG, Edwards BK (eds). SEER Cancer Statistics Review, 1975-2007, National Cancer Institute. Bethesda, MD, http://seer.cancer.gov/csr/1975_2007/, based on November 2009 SEER data submission, posted to the SEER web site, 2010

Ford D, Easton DF, Bishop DT, et al. Risks of cancer in BRCA1-mutation carriers. Breast Cancer Linkage Consortium. Lancet 1994;343:692-5.

Liede A, Karlan BY, Narod SA. Cancer risks for male carriers of germline mutations in BRCA1 or BRCA2: a review of the literature.

Wooster R, Neuhausen SL, Mangion J, et al. Localization of a breast cancer susceptibility gene, BRCA2, to chromosome 13q12-13. Science 1994;265:2088-90.

Page DL, Dupont WD, Rogers LW, Rados MS. Atypical ductal hyperplastic lesions of the female breast. A long-term follow-up study. Cancer 1985;55:2698-708.

Dixon JM, McDonald C, Elton RA, Miller WR. Risk of breast cancer in women with palpable breast cysts: a prospective study. Edinburgh Breast Group. Lancet 1999; 353:1742-5.

Collaborative Group on Hormonal Factors in Breast Cancer. Familial breast cancer: col-laborative reanalysis of individual data from 52 epidemiological studies including 58,209 women with breast cancer and 101,986 women without the disease. Lancet 2001;358:1389-99.

Breast. In: Edge SB, Byrd DR, Compton CC, eds. *AJCC Cancer Staging Manual.* 7th ed. New York, NY: Springer, 2010, pp. 347-67.

Saslow D, Boetes C, Burke W, et al. American Cancer Society guidelines for breast screening with MRI as an adjunct to mammography. CA Cancer J Clin 2007;57:75-89.

Lord SJ, Lei W, Craft P, et al. A systematic review of the effectiveness of magnetic resonance imaging (MRI) as an addition to mammography and ultrasound in screening young women at high risk of breast cancer. Eur J Cancer 2007;43:1905-17.

Houssami N, Ciatto S, Macaskill P, et al. Accuracy and surgical impact of magnetic resonance imaging in breast cancer staging: systematic review and meta-analysis in detection of multifocal and multicentric cancer. J Clin Oncol 2008;26:3248-58.

Turnbull L. Magnetic resonance imaging in breast cancer: results of the COMICE trial. Breast Cancer Res 2008;10:10.

Houssami N, Hayes DF. Review of preoperative magnetic resonance imaging (MRI) in breast cancer: Should MRI be performed on all women with newly diagnosed, early stage breast cancer? CA Cancer J Clin 2009;59:290-302.

Brennan ME, Houssami N, Lord S, et al. Magnetic resonance imaging screening of the contralateral breast in women with newly diagnosed breast cancer: systematic review and meta-analysis of incremental cancer detection and impact on surgical management. J Clin Oncol 2009;27:5640-9.

Mamounas EP, Tang G, Fisher B, et al. Association between the 21-gene Recurrence Score assay and risk of locoregional recurrence in node-negative, estrogen receptor-positive breast cancer: results from NSABP B-14 and NSABP B-20. J Clin Oncol 2010; 28:1677-83.

Dowsett M, Cuzick J, Wale C, et al. Prediction of distant recurrence using the 21-gene Recurrence Score in node-negative and node-positive postmenopausal patients with breast cancer treated with anastrazole or tamoxifen: a TransATAC study. J Clin Oncol 2010;28:1829-34.

Lo SS, Mumby PB, Norton J, et al. Prospective multicenter study of the impact of the 21-gene Recurrence Score assay on medical oncologist and patient adjuvant breast cancer treatment selection. J Clin Oncol 2010;28:1671-6.

Fisher B, Anderson S, Bryant J, et al. Twenty-year follow-up of a randomized trial comparing total mastectomy, lumpectomy, and lumpectomy plus irradiation for the treatment of invasive breast cancer. N Eng J Med 2002;347:1233-41.

Fisher B, Jeong JH, Anderson S, et al. Twenty-five year follow-up of a randomized trial comparing radical mastectomy, total mastectomy, and total mastectomy followed by irradiation. N Eng J Med 2002;347:567-75.

Veronesi U, Cascinelli N, Mariani L, et al. Twenty-year follow-up of a randomized study comparing breast-conserving surgery with radical mastectomy for early stage breast cancer. N Eng J Med 2002;347:1227-32.

Fyles AW, McCready DR, Manchul LA, et al. Tamoxifen with or without breast irradiation in women 50 years of age or older with early breast cancer. N Eng J Med 2004; 351:963-70.

Early Breast Cancer Trialists' Collaborative Group. Effects of radiotherapy and of differences in the extent of surgery for early breast cancer on local recurrence and 15-year survival: an overview of the randomized trials. Lancet 2005;366:2087-2106.

Hughes KS, Schnaper LA, Berry D, et al. Lumpectomy plus tamoxifen with or without irradiation in women 70 years of age or older with early breast cancer. N Eng J Med 2004;351:951-977.

START Trialists' Group, Bentzen SM, Agrawal RK, Aird EG, et al. The UK Standardization of Breast Radiotherapy (START) Trial A of radiotherapy hypofractionation for treatment of early breast cancer: a randomized trial. Lancet Oncol 2008;9:331-41.

START Trialists' Group, Bentzen SM, Agrawal RK, Aird EG, et al. The UK Standardization of Breast Radiotherapy (START) Trial B of radiotherapy hypofractionation for treatment of early breast cancer: a randomized trial. Lancet 2008;371:1098-1107.

Whelan TJ, Pignol JP, Levine MN, et al. Long-term results of hypofractionated radiation therapy for breast cancer. N Eng J Med 2010;362:513-20.

Overgaard M, Hansen PS, Overgaard J, et al. Postoperative radiotherapy on high-risk premenopausal women with breast cancer who receive adjuvant chemotherapy. Danish Breast Cancer Cooperative Group 82b Trial. N Eng J Med 1997;337:949-55.

Ragaz J, Jackson SM, Le N, et al. Adjuvant radiotherapy and chemotherapy in node-positive premenopausal women with breast cancer. N Eng J Med 1997;337:956-62.

Overgaard M, Jensen MB, Overgaard J, et al. Postoperative radiotherapy in high-risk postmenopausal breast-cancer patients given adjuvant tamoxifen: Danish Breast Cancer Cooperative Group DBCG 82c randomized trial. Lancet 1999;353:1641-8.

Ragaz J, Olivotto IA, Spinelli JJ, et al. Locoregional radiation therapy in patients with high-risk breast cancer receiving adjuvant chemotherapy: 20-year results if the British Columbia randomized trial. J Natl Cancer Inst 2005;97:116-26.

Ernster VL, Barclay J, Kerlikowske K, et al. Incidence of and treatment for ductal carcinoma in situ of the breast. JAMA 1996;275:913-8.

Fisher B, Dignam J, Wolmark N, et al. Lumpectomy and radiation therapy for the treatment of intraductal breast cancer: findings from the National Surgical Adjuvant Breast and Bowel Project B-17. J Clin Oncol 1998;16:441-52.

Silverstein MJ, Lagos MD, Groshen S, et al. The influence of margin width on local control of ductal carcinoma in situ. N Eng J Med 1999;340:1455-61.

Houghton J, George WD, Cuzick J, et al. Radiotherapy and tamoxifen in women with completely excised ductal carcinoma in situ of the breast in the UK, Australia, and New Zealand: a randomized trial. Lancet 2003;362:95-102.

Bijker N, Meijnen P, Peterse JL, et al. Breast-conserving treatment with or without radiotherapy in ductal carcinoma-in-situ: ten-year results of the European Organization for Research and Treatment of Cancer randomized phase III trial 10853—a study by the EORTC Breast Cancer Cooperative Group and EORTC Radiotherapy Group. J Clin Oncol 2006;24:3381-7.

Hughes LL, Wang M, Page DL, et al. Local excision alone without irradiation for ductal carcinoma in situ of the breast: a trial of the Eastern Cooperative Oncology Group. J Clin Oncol 2009;27:5319-24.

Arthur DW, Vicini FA, Kuske RR, et al. Accelerated partial breast irradiation: an updated report from the American Brachytherapy Society. Brachytherapy 2003;2:124-30.

Vicini F, Beitsch P, Quiet C, et al. Five-year analysis of treatment efficacy and cosmesis by the American Society of Breast Surgeons MammoSite Breast Brachytherapy Registry Trial in patients treated with accelerated breast irradiation. Int J Radiat Oncol Biol Phys 2010; May 14 [Epub ahead of print].

Shaitelman SF, Vicini FA, Beitsch P, et al. Five-year outcome of patients classified using the American Society for Radiation Oncology consensus statement guidelines for the application of accelerated partial breast irradiation: an analysis of patients treated on the American Society of Breast Surgeons MammoSite Registry Trial. Cancer 2010, July 2 [Epub ahead of print].

Paik S, Bryant J, Park C, et al. erbB-2 and response to doxorubicin in patients with axillary lymph node-positive, hormone receptor-negative breast cancer. J Natl Cancer Inst 1998;90:1361-70.

Colleoni M, Cole BF, Viale G, et al. Classical cyclophosphamide, methotrexate, and fluorouracil chemotherapy is more effective in triple-negative, node-negative breast cancer: results from two randomized trials of adjuvant chemoendocrine therapy for node-negative breast cancer. J Clin Oncol 2010;28:2966-70.

Early Breast Cancer Trialists' Collaborative Group. Effects of chemotherapy and hormonal therapy for early breast cancer on local recurrence and 15-year survival: an overview of the randomized trials. Lancet 2005;366:1687-1717.

Bellon JR, Come SE, Gelman RS, et al. Sequencing of chemotherapy and radiation therapy in early-stage breast cancer: updated results of a prospective randomized trial. J Clin Oncol 2005;23:1934-40.

Early Breast Cancer Trialists' Collaborative Group. Polychemotherapy for early breast cancer: an overview of the randomized trials. Lancet 1998; 352:930-42.

Early Breast Cancer Trialists' Collaborative Group. Tamoxifen for early breast cancer: an overview of the randomized trials. Lancet 1998; 351:1451-67.

Fisher B, Cosantino J, Redmond C, et al. A randomized clinical trial evaluating tamoxifen in the treatment of patients with node-negative breast cancer who have estrogen-receptor positive tumors. N Eng J Med 1989;320:479-484.

Fisher B, Cosantino JP, Wickerham DL, et al. Tamoxifen for prevention of breast cancer: current status of the National Surgical Adjuvant Breast and Bowel Project P-1 Study. J Natl Cancer Inst 2005;97:1652-62.

Fisher B, Bryant J, Dignam JL, et al. Tamoxifen, radiation therapy, or both for prevention of ipsilateral breast tumor recurrence after lumpectomy in women with invasive breast cancers of one centimeter or less. N Eng J Med 2002;20:4141-9.

Fisher B, Dignam J, Wolmark N, et al. Tamoxifen in treatment of intraductal breast cancer: National Surgical Adjuvant Breast and Bowel Project B-24 randomized controlled trial. Lancet 1999;353:1993-2000.

Dowsett M, Cuzick J, Coates A, et al. Meta-analysis of breast cancer outcomes in adjuvant trials of aromatase inhibitors versus tamoxifen. J Clin Oncol 2010;28:509-18.

Slamon DJ, Leyland-Jones B, Shak S, et al. Use of chemotherapy plus a monoclonal antibody against HER2 for metastatic breast cancer that overexpresses HER2. N Eng J Med 2001;344:783-92.

Romond EH, Perez EA, Bryant J, et al. Trastuzumab plus adjuvant chemotherapy for operable HER2-positive breast cancer. N Eng J Med 2005;353:1673-84.

Piccart-Gebhart MJ, Procter M, Leyland-Jones B, et al. Trastuzumab after adjuvant chemotherapy in HER2-positive breast cancer. N Eng J Med 2005;353:1659-72.

Smith I, Procter M, Gelber RD, et al. 2-year follow-up of trastuzumab after adjuvant chemotherapy in HER2-positive breast cancer: a randomized controlled trial. Lancet 2007;369:29-36.

Gianni L, Eiermann W, Semiglazov V, et al. Neoadjuvant chemotherapy with trastuzumab followed by adjuvant trastuzumab versus neoadjuvant chemotherapy alone, in patients with HER2-positive locally advanced breast cancer (the NOAH trial): a randomized controlled superiority trial with a parallel NER2-negative cohort.

Rennert G, Pinchev M, Rennert H. Use of bisphosphonates and risk of postmenopausal breast cancer. J Clin Oncol 2010;28:3577—81.

Chlebowski RT, Chen Z, Cauley J, et al. Oral bisphosphonate use and breast cancer incidence in postmenopausal women. J Clin Oncol 2010;28:3582-90.

COLORECTAL CANCER

Altekruse SF, Kosary CL, Krapcho M, Neyman N, Aminou R, Waldron W, Ruhl J, Howlader N, Tatalovich Z, Cho H, Mariotto A, Eisner MP, Lewis DR, Cronin K, Chen HS, Feuer EJ, Stinchcomb DG, Edwards BK (eds). SEER Cancer Statistics Review, 1975-2007, National Cancer Institute. Bethesda, MD, http://seer.cancer.gov/csr/1975_2007/, based on November 2009 SEER data submission, posted to the SEER web site, 2010

Myerson RJ, Colon and rectum. In: Perez CA, Brady LW, Halperin EC, et al., editors. Principles and Practice of Radiation Oncology. 4th ed. Philadelphia: Lippincott Williams and Wilkins; 2004. pp. 1607-1629.

Colon and Rectum. In: Edge SB, Byrd DR, Compton CC, eds. *AJCC Cancer Staging Manual.* 7th ed. New York, NY: Springer, 2010, pp. 143-64.

Gunderson LL, Sargent DJ, Tepper JE, et al. Impact of T and N stage and treatment on survival and relapse in adjuvant rectal cancer: a pooled analysis. Int J Radiat Oncol Biol Phys 2002;22:1785-96.

Moertel CG, Fleming TR, MacDonald JS, et al. Levamisole and fluorouracil for adjuvant therapy of resected colon carcinoma. N Eng J Med 1990;322:352-8.

Haller DG, Catalano PJ, MacDonald JS, et al. Phase III study of fluorouracil, leucovorin, and levamisole in high-risk stage II and III colon cancer: final report of Intergroup 0089. J Clin Oncol 2005;23:8671-8.

Andre T, Boni C, Mounedji-Boudiaf L, et al. Oxaliplatin, fluorouracil, and leucovorin as adjuvant treatment for colon cancer. N Eng J Med 2004;350:2353-51. .

Andre T, Boni C, Navarro M, et al. Improved overall survival with oxaliplatin, fluorouracil, and leucovorin as adjuvant treatment in stage II and III colon cancer in the MOSAIC trial. J Clin Oncol 2009;27:3109-16.

Krook JE, Moertel CG, Gunderson LL, et al. Effective surgical adjuvant therapy for high-risk rectal carcinoma. N Eng J Med 1991;324:709-15.

O'Connell MJ, Martenson JA, Wieand HS, et al. Improving adjuvant therapy for rectal cancer by combining protracted-infusion fluorouracil with radiation therapy after curative surgery. N Eng J Med 1994;331:502-7.

[No authors listed] Improved survival with preoperative radiotherapy in resectable rectal cancer. Swedish Rectal Cancer Trial. N Eng J Med 1997;336:980-7.

Kapiteijn E, Marijnen CA, Nagtegaal ID, et al. Preoperative radiotherapy combined with total mesorectal excision for resectable rectal cancer. N Eng J Med 2001; 345:638-46.

Sauer R, Becker H, Hohenberger W, et al. Preoperative versus postoperative chemoradiotherapy for rectal cancer. N Eng J Med 2004;351:1731-40.

Roh MS, Colangelo LH, O'Connell MJ, et al. Preoperative multimodality therapy improves disease free survival in patients with carcinoma of the rectum: NSABP R-03. J Clin Oncol 2009;27:5124-31.

Goldberg RM, Sargent DJ, Morton RF, et al. Randomized controlled trial of reduced-dose bolus fluorouracil plus leucovorin and irinotecan or infused fluorouracil plus leucovorin and oxaliplatin in patients with previously untreated metastatic colorectal cancer: a North American Intergroup Trial. J Clin Oncol 2006;24:3347-53.

Hurwitz H, Fehrenbacher L, Novotny W, et al. Bevacizumab plus irinotecan, fluorouracil, and leucovorin for metastatic colorectal cancer. N Eng J Med 2004;350:2335-42.

Saltz LB, Clarke S, Diaz-Rubio E, et al. Bevacizumab in combination with oxaliplatin-based chemotherapy as first-line therapy in metastatic colorectal cancer: a randomized phase III study. J Clin Oncol 2008;26:2013-9.

Fong Y, Cohen AM, Fortner JG, et al. Liver resection for colorectal metastases. J Clin Oncol 1997;15:938-46.

Choti MA, Sitzmann JV, Tiburi MF et al. Trends in long-term survival following liver resection for hepatic colorectal metastases. Ann Surg 2002;235:759-66.

Minagawa M, Yamamoto J, Miwa S, et al. Selection criteria for simultaneous resection in patients with synchronous liver metastasis. Arch Surg 2006;141:1006-12.

Nguyen KT, Laurent A, Dagher I, et al. Minimally invasive liver resection for metastatic colorectal cancer: a multi-institutional, international report of safety, feasibility, and early outcomes. Ann Surg 2009;250:842-8.

Nordlinger B, Sorbye H, Glimelius B, et al. Perioperative chemotherapy with FOLFOX4 and surgery versus surgery alone for resectable liver metastases from colorectal cancer (EORTC Intergroup trial 40983): a randomized controlled trial. Lancet 2008; 371:1007-16.

Gillams AR, Lees WR. Radiofrequency ablation of colorectal liver metastases in 167 patients. Eur Radiol 2004;14:2261-7.

Chen MH, Yang W, Yan K, et al. Treatment efficacy of radiofrequency ablation of 338 patients with hepatic malignant tumor and the relevant complications. World J Gastroenterol 2005;11:6395-6401.

Machi J, Oishi AJ, Sumida K, et al. Long-term outcome of radiofrequency ablation for unresectable liver metastases from colorectal cancer: Evaluation of prognostic factors and effectiveness in first- and second-line management. Cancer J 2006;12:318-26.

Wong SL, Mangu PB, Choti MA, et al. American Society of Clinical Oncology 2009 clinical evidence review on radiofrequency ablation of hepatic metastases from colorectal cancer. J Clin Oncol 2010;28:493-508.

Hendlisz A, Van den Eynde M, Peeters M, et al. Phase III trial comparing protracted intravenous fluorouracil infusion alone or with Yttrium-90 resin microspheres radioembolization for liver-limited metastatic colorectal cancer refractory to standard chemotherapy. J Clin Oncol 2010;28:3687-94.

ESOPHAGEAL CANCER

Altekruse SF, Kosary CL, Krapcho M, Neyman N, Aminou R, Waldron W, Ruhl J, Howlader N, Tatalovich Z, Cho H, Mariotto A, Eisner MP, Lewis DR, Cronin K, Chen HS, Feuer EJ, Stinchcomb DG, Edwards BK (eds). SEER Cancer Statistics Review, 1975-2007, National Cancer Institute. Bethesda, MD, http://seer.cancer.gov/csr/1975_2007/, based on November 2009 SEER data submission, posted to the SEER web site, 2010

Esophagus and Esophagogastric Junction. In: Edge SB, Byrd DR, Compton CC, eds. *AJCC Cancer Staging Manual.* 7th ed. New York, NY: Springer, 2010, pp. 103-116.

Hong D, Lunagomez S, Kim EE, et al. Value of baseline positron emission tomography for predicting overall survival in patients with nonmetastatic esophageal or gastroesophageal junction carcinoma. Cancer 2006;104:1620-6.

Swisher SG, Erasmus J, Maish M, et al. 2-fluoro-2-deoxy-D-glucose positron emission tomography imaging is predictive of pathologic response and survival after preoperative chemoradiation in patients with esophageal carcinoma. Cancer 2004;101:1776-85.

Kaushik N, Khalid A, Brody D, et al. Endoscopic ultrasound compared with laparoscopy for staging esophageal cancer. Ann Thorac Surg 2007;83:2000-2.

Visbal AL, Allen MS, Miller DL, et al. Ivor Lewis esophagogastrectomy for esophageal cancer. Ann Thorac Surg 2001;71:1803-8.

Atkins BZ, Shah AS, Hutcheson KA, et al. Reducing hospital morbidity and mortality following esophagectomy. Ann Thorac Surg 2004;78:1170-6.

Cooper JS, Guo MD, Herskovic A, et al. Chemoradiotherapy of locally advanced esophageal cancer: long-term follow-up of a prospective randomized trial (RTOG 85-01). JAMA 1999;281:1623-7.

Minsky BD, Pajak TF, Ginsberg RJ, et al. INT 0123 (Radiation Therapy Oncology Group 94-05) phase III trial of combined modality therapy for esophageal cancer: high-dose versus standard-dose radiation therapy. J Clin Oncol 2002;20:1167-1174.

Walsh TN, Noonan N, Hollywood D, et al. A comparison of multimodal therapy and surgery for esophageal adenocarcinoma. N Eng J Med 1996;335:462-7.

HEAD & NECK CANCER

Altekruse SF, Kosary CL, Krapcho M, Neyman N, Aminou R, Waldron W, Ruhl J, Howlader N, Tatalovich Z, Cho H, Mariotto A, Eisner MP, Lewis DR, Cronin K, Chen HS, Feuer EJ, Stinchcomb DG, Edwards BK (eds). SEER Cancer Statistics Review, 1975-2007, National Cancer Institute. Bethesda, MD, http://seer.cancer.gov/csr/1975_2007/, based on November 2009 SEER data submission, posted to the SEER web site, 2010

Lip and Oral Cavity. In: Edge SB, Byrd DR, Compton CC, eds. *AJCC Cancer Staging Manual.* 7th ed. New York, NY: Springer, 2010, pp. 29-40.

Pharynx. In: Edge SB, Byrd DR, Compton CC, eds. *AJCC Cancer Staging Manual.* 7th ed. New York, NY: Springer, 2010, pp. 41-56.

Larynx. In: Edge SB, Byrd DR, Compton CC, eds. *AJCC Cancer Staging Manual.* 7th ed. New York, NY: Springer, 2010, pp. 57-68.

Fakhry C, Westra WH, Li S, et al. Improved survival of patients with human papillomavirus positive head and neck squamous cell carcinoma in a prospective clinical trial. J Natl Cancer Inst 2008;100:261-9.

Gillison M, D'Souza G, Westra W, et al. Distinct risk factor profiles for human papillomavirus type 16-positive and human papillomavirus 16-negative head and neck cancers. J Natl Cancer Inst 2008;100:407-20.

Ang KK, Harris J, Wheeler R, et al. Human papillomavirus and survival of patients with oropharyngeal cancer. N Eng J Med 363:24-35.

Lin JC, Wang WY, Chen KY, et al. Quantification of plasma Epstein-Barr virus DNA in patients with advanced nasopharyngeal carcinoma. N Eng J Med 2004;350:2461-70.

Lonneux M, Hamoir M, Reychler H, et al. Positron emission tomography with [18F] fluorodeoxyglucose improves staging and patient management in patients with head and neck squamous cell carcinoma: a multicenter prospective study. J Clin Oncol 2010;28:1190-5.

Bernier J, Domenge C, Ozsahin M, et al. Postoperative irradiation with or without concomitant chemotherapy for locally advanced head and neck cancer. N Eng J Med 2004;350:1945-52.

Cooper JS, Pajak TF, Forastiere AA, et al. Postoperative concurrent radiotherapy and chemotherapy for high-risk squamous-cell carcinoma of the head and neck. N Eng J Med 2004;350:1937-44.

Horiot JC, Bontemps P, van den Bogaert W, et al. Accelerated fractionation (AF) compared to conventional fractionation (CF) improves locoregional control in the radiotherapy of advanced head and neck cancers: results of the EORTC 22851 randomized trial. Radiother Oncol 1997;44:111-21.

Bourhis J, Overgaard J, Audry H, et al. Hyperfractionated or accelerated radiotherapy in head and neck cancer: a meta-analysis. Lancet 2006 368:843-54.

[No authors listed] Induction chemotherapy plus radiation compared with surgery plus radiation in patients with advanced laryngeal cancer. The Department of Veterans Affairs Laryngeal Cancer Study Group. N Eng J Med 1991;324:1685-90.

Lefebvre JL, Chevalier D, Luboinski B, et al. Larynx preservation in pyriform sinus cancer: preliminary results of a European Organization for Research and Treatment of Cancer phase III trial. EORTC Head and Neck Cancer Cooperative Group. J Natl Cancer Inst 1996;88:890-9.

Al-Sarraf M, LeBlanc M, Girl PG, et al. Chemoradiotherapy versus radiotherapy in patients with advanced nasopharyngeal cancer: phase III randomized Intergroup study 0099. J Clin Oncol 1998;16:1310-7.

Brizel DM, Albers ME, Fisher SR, et al. Hyperfractionated irradiation with or without concurrent chemotherapy for locally advanced head and neck cancer. N Eng J Med 1998;338:1798-1804.

Adelstein DJ, Li Y, Adams GL, et al. An intergroup phase III comparison of standard radiation therapy and two schedules of concurrent chemoradiotherapy in patients with unresectable squamous cell head and neck cancer. J Clin Oncol 2003; 21:92-8.

Denis F, Garaud P, Bardet E, et al. Final results of the 94-01 French Head and Neck Oncology and Radiotherapy Group randomized trial comparing radiotherapy alone with concomitant radiochemotherapy in advanced-stage oropharyngeal cancer. J Clin Oncol 2004;22:69-76.

Forastiere AA, Goepfert H, Maor M, et al. Concurrent chemotherapy and radiotherapy for organ preservation in advanced laryngeal cancer. N Eng J Med 2003;349:2091-8.

Pignon JP, le Maitre A, Maillard E, et al. Meta-analysis of chemotherapy in head and neck cancer (MACH-NC): an update on 93 randomized trials and 17,346 patients. Radiother Oncol 2009;92:4-14.

Bonner JA, Harari PM, Giralt J, et al. Radiotherapy plus cetuximab for squamous-cell carcinoma of the head and neck. N Eng J Med 2006;354:567-78.

Vermorken JB, Mesia R, Rivera F, et al. Platinum-based chemotherapy plus cetuximab in head and neck cancer. N Eng J Med 2008;359:1116-27.

Bonner JA, Harari PM, Giralt J, et al. Radiotherapy plus cetuximab for locoregionally advanced head and neck cancer: 5-year survival data from a phase 3 randomized trial, and relation between cetuximab-induced rash and survival. Lancet Oncol 2010;11:21-8.

Remmier D, Byers R, Scheetz, et al. A prospective study of shoulder disability resulting from radical and modified radical neck dissections. Head Neck Surg 1986;8:280-6.

Terrell JE, Welsh DE, Bradford CR, et al. Pain, quality of life, and spinal accessory nerve status after neck dissection. Laryngoscope 2000;110:620-6.

Clayman GL, Johnson CJ, Morrison W, et al. The role of neck dissection after chemoradiotherapy for oropharyngeal cancer with advanced nodal disease. Arch Otolaryngol Head Neck Surg 2001;127:135-9.

Lango MN, Myers JN, Garden AS. Controversies in surgical management of the node-positive neck after chemoradiation. Semin Radiat Oncol 2009;19:24-8.

Van der Putten L, van den Broek GB, de Bree R, et al. Effectiveness of salvage selective and modified radical neck dissection for regional pathologic lymphadenopathy after chemoradiation. Head Neck 2009;31:593-603.

KIDNEY CANCER

Altekruse SF, Kosary CL, Krapcho M, Neyman N, Aminou R, Waldron W, Ruhl J, Howlader N, Tatalovich Z, Cho H, Mariotto A, Eisner MP, Lewis DR, Cronin K, Chen HS, Feuer EJ, Stinchcomb DG, Edwards BK (eds). SEER Cancer Statistics Review, 1975-2007, National Cancer Institute. Bethesda, MD, http://seer.cancer.gov/csr/1975_2007/, based on November 2009 SEER data submission, posted to the SEER web site, 2010

Kidney. In: Edge SB, Byrd DR, Compton CC, eds. AJCC Cancer Staging Manual. 7th ed. New York, NY: Springer, 2010, pp. 479-90.

Levine E. Renal cell carcinoma in uremic acquired renal cystic disease: incidence, detection, and management. Urol Radiol 1992;13:203-10.

Pavlovich CP, Schmidt LS, Phillips JL. The genetic basis of renal cell carcinoma. Urol Clin North Am 2003;30:437-54.

Clark PE, Cookson MS. The von Hippel-Lindau gene: turning discovery onto therapy. Cancer 2008;113:1768-78.

Ghavamian R, Cheville JC, Lohse CM, et al. Renal cell carcinoma in the solitary kidney: an analysis of complications and outcome after nephron sparing surgery. J Urol 2002;168:454-9.

Brandina R, Aron M. Laparoscopic partial nephrectomy: advances since 2005. Curr Opin Urol 2010;20:111-8.

Cowey CL, Hutson TE. Molecularly targeted agents for renal cell carcinoma: the next generation. Clin Adv Hematol Oncol 2010;8:357-64.

Escudier B, Eisen T, Stadler WM, et al. Sorafenib in advanced clear-cell renal-cell carcinoma. N Eng J Med 2007;356:125-34.

Motzer RJ, Hutson TE, Tomczak P, et al. Overall survival and updated results for sunitinib compared with interferon alpha in patients with metastatic renal cell carcinoma. J Clin Oncol 2009;27:3584-90.

Sternberg CN, Davis ID, Mardiak J, et al. Pazopanib in locally advanced or metastatic renal cell carcinoma: results of a randomized phase III trial. J Clin Oncol 2010;28:1061-8.

Hudes G, Carducci M, Tomczak P, et al. Temsirolimus, interferon alpha, or both for advanced renal-cell carcinoma. N Eng J med 2007;356:2271-81.

Motzer RJ, Escudier B, Oudard S, et al. Efficacy of everolimus in advanced renal cell carcinoma: a double-blind, randomized, placebo-controlled phase III trial. Lancet 2008;372:449-56.

Yang JC, Haworth L, Sherry RM, et al. A randomized trial of bevacizumab, an anti-vascular endothelial growth factor antibody, for metastatic renal cancer. N Eng J Med 2003;349:427-34.

Escudier B, Bellmunt J, Negrier S, et al. Phase III trial of bevacizumab plus interferon alfa-2a in patients with metastatic renal cell carcinoma (AVOREN): final analysis of overall survival. J Clin Oncol 2010;28:2144-50.

Rini BI, Halabi S, Rosenberg JE, et al. Phase III trial of bevacizumab plus interferon alfa versus interferon alfa monotherapy in patients with metastatic renal cell carcinoma: final results of CALGB 90206. J Clin Oncol 2010;28:2137-43.

LEUKEMIA

Altekruse SF, Kosary CL, Krapcho M, Neyman N, Aminou R, Waldron W, Ruhl J, Howlader N, Tatalovich Z, Cho H, Mariotto A, Eisner MP, Lewis DR, Cronin K, Chen HS, Feuer EJ, Stinchcomb DG, Edwards BK (eds). SEER Cancer Statistics Review, 1975-2007,

National Cancer Institute. Bethesda, MD, http://seer.cancer.gov/csr/1975_2007/, based on November 2009 SEER data submission, posted to the SEER web site, 2010

Johnson S, Smith AG, Loffler H, et al. Multicentre prospective randomized trial of fludarabine versus cyclophosphamide, doxorubicin, and prednisone (CAP) for treatment of advanced-stage chronic lymphocytic leukaemia. The French Cooperative Group on CLL. Lancet 1996;347:1432-8.

Keating MJ, O'Brien S, Lerner S, et al. Long-term follow-up of patients with chronic lymphocytic leukemia (CLL) receiving fludarabine regimens as initial therapy. Blood 1998;92:1165-71.

Schriever F, Huhn D. New directions on the diagnosis and treatment of chronic lymphocytic leukaemia. Drugs 2003;63:953-69.

Knauf WU, Lissichov T, Aldaoud A, et al. Phase III randomized study of bendamustine compared with chlorambucil in previously untreated patients with chronic lymphocytic leukemia. J Clin Oncol 2009;27:4378-84.

Jabbour EJ, Estey E, Kantarjian HM. Adult acute myeloid leukemia. Mayo Clin Proc 2006;81:247-60.

Brunning RD, Matutes E, Harris NL, et al. Acute myeloid leukaemia: introduction. In: Jaffe ES, Harris NL, Stein H, et al., eds.: Pathology and Genetics of Tumours of Haematopoietic Lymphoid Tissues. Lyon, France: IARC Press, 2001. World Health Organization Classification of Tumours, 3:77-80.

Wiernik PH, Banks PL, Case DC, et al. Cytarabine plus idarubicin or daunorubicin as induction and consolidation therapy for previously untreated adult patients with acute myeloid leukemia. Blood 1992;79:313-9.

Vogler WR, Velez-Garcia E, Weiner RS, et al. A phase III trial comparing idarubicin and daunorubicin in combination with cytarabine in acute myelogenous leukemia: a Southeastern Cancer Study Group Study. J Clin Oncol 1992;10:1103-11.

Mayer RJ, Davis RB, Schiffer CA, et al. Intensive postremission chemotherapy in adults with acute myeloid leukemia. Cancer and Leukemia Group B. N Eng J Med 1994;331:896-903.

Casileth PA, Harrington DP, Applebaum FR, et al. Chemotherapy compared with autologous or allogeneic bone marrow transplantation in the management of acute myeloid leukemia in first remission. N Eng J Med 1998;339:1649-56.

Grinwade D, Walker H, Harrison G, et al. The predictive value of hierarchical cytogenetic classification in older adults with acute myeloid leukemia (AML): analysis of 1065 patients entered into the United Kingdom Medical Research Council AML11 trial. Blood 2001;98:1312-20.

Sokal JE, Cox EB, Baccarani M, et al. Prognostic discrimination in "good-risk" chronic granulocytic leukemia. Blood 1984;63:789-99.

O'Brien SG, Guilhot F, Larson RA, et al. Imatinib compared with interferon and low-dose cytarabine for newly diagnosed chronic phase chronic myeloid leukemia. N Eng J Med 2003;348:994-1004.

Hughes TP, Kaeda J, Branford S, et al. Frequency of major molecular responses to imatinib or interferon alpha plus cytarabine in newly diagnosed chronic myeloid leukemia. N Eng J Med 2003;349:1423-32.

Baccarani M, Cortes J, Pane F, et al. Chronic myeloid leukemia: an update of concepts and management recommendations of European LeukemiaNet. J Clin Oncol 2009; 27:6041-51.

Saglio G, Kim DW, Issararisil S, et al. Nilotinib versus imatinib for newly diagnosed chromic myeloid leukemia. N Eng J Med 2010;362:2251-9.

Kantarjian H, Shah N, Hochhaus A, et al. Dasatinib versus imatinib in newly diagnosed chronic-phase chronic myeloid leukemia. N Eng J Med 2010;362:2260-70.

Copelan EA, McGuire EA. The biology and treatment of acute lymphoblastic leukemia in adults. Blood 1995;85:1151-68.

LIVER CANCERS

Altekruse SF, Kosary CL, Krapcho M, Neyman N, Aminou R, Waldron W, Ruhl J, Howlader N, Tatalovich Z, Cho H, Mariotto A, Eisner MP, Lewis DR, Cronin K, Chen HS, Feuer EJ, Stinchcomb DG, Edwards BK (eds). SEER Cancer Statistics Review, 1975-2007, National Cancer Institute. Bethesda, MD, http://seer.cancer.gov/csr/1975_2007/, based on November 2009 SEER data submission, posted to the SEER web site, 2010.

Schafer DF, Sorrell MF. Hepatocellular carcinoma. Lancet 1999;353:1253-7.

El-Serag HB. Hepatocellular carcinoma and hepatitis C in the United States. Hepatology 2002;36:S74-83.

El-Serag HB. Hepatocellular carcinoma: recent trends in the United States. Gastroenterology 2004;127:S27-34.

Liver. In: Edge SB, Byrd DR, Compton CC, eds. *AJCC Cancer Staging Manual.* 7th ed. New York, NY: Springer, 2010, pp. 191-200.

Child CG, Turcotte JG. Surgery and portal hypertension. In: The liver and portal hypertension. Edited by CG Child. Philadelphia: Saunders 1964:50-64.

Pugh RN, Murray-Lyon IM, Dawson JL, et al. Transection of the oesophagus for bleeding oesophageal varices. B J Surg 1973;60:646-9.

Kamath PS, Kim WR. The model for end-stage liver disease (MELD) Hepatology 2007;45:797-805.

Llovet JM, Burroughs A, Bruix J. Hepatocellular carcinoma. Lancet 2003;362:1907-17.

Poon RT, Fan ST, Lo CM, et al. Long-term survival and pattern of recurrence after resection of small hepatocellular carcinoma in patients with preserved liver function: implications for a strategy of salvage transplantation. Ann Surg 2002;235:373-82.

Morris-Stiff G, Gomez D, de Ligouri CN, Prasad KR. Surgical management of hepatocellular carcinoma: is the jury still out? Surg Oncol 2009;18:298-321.

Nathan H, Schulick RD, Choti MA, Pawlik TM. Predictors of survival after resection of hepatocellular carcinoma. Ann Surg 2009;249:799-805.

Schwartz RE, Smith DD. Trends in local therapy for hepatocellular carcinoma and survival outcomes in the U.S. population. Am J Surg 2008;195:829-36.

Yeh CN, Chen MF, Lee WC, Jeng LB. Prognostic factors of hepatic resection for hepatocellular carcinoma with cirrhosis: univariate and multivariate analysis. J Surg Oncol 2002;81:195-202.

Lin SM, Lin CJ, Hsu CW, Chen YC. Radiofrequency ablation improves prognosis compared with ethanol injection for hepatocellular carcinoma < or =4 cm. Gastroenterology 2004;127:1714-23.

Zhou WP, Lai EC, Li AJ, et al. A prospective, randomized, controlled trial of preoperative transarterial chemoembolization for resectable large hepatocellular carcinoma. Ann Surg 2009;249:195-202.

Cheng BQ, Jia CQ, Liu CT, et al. Chemoembolization combined with radiofrequency ablation for patients with hepatocellular carcinoma larger than 3 cm: a randomized controlled trial. JAMA 2008;299:1669-7

LUNG CANCER

Altekruse SF, Kosary CL, Krapcho M, Neyman N, Aminou R, Waldron W, Ruhl J, Howlader N, Tatalovich Z, Cho H, Mariotto A, Eisner MP, Lewis DR, Cronin K, Chen HS, Feuer EJ, Stinchcomb DG, Edwards BK (eds). SEER Cancer Statistics Review, 1975-2007,

National Cancer Institute. Bethesda, MD, http://seer.cancer.gov/csr/1975_2007/, based on November 2009 SEER data submission, posted to the SEER web site, 2010.

Sculier JP, Chansky K, Crowley JJ, et al. The impact of additional prognostic factors on survival and their relationship with the anatomical extent of disease expressed by the 6th Edition of the TNM Classification of Malignant Tumors and the proposals for the 7th Edition. J Thorac Oncol 2008;3:457-66.

Slatore CG, Chien JW, Au DH, et al. Lung cancer and hormone replacement therapy: association in the Vitamins and Lifestyle Study. J Clin Oncol 2010;28:15406.

Chlebowski RT, Schwartz AG, Wakelee H, et al. Oestrogen plus progestin and lung cancer in postmenopausal women (Women's Health Initiative trial): a post-hoc analysis of a randomized controlled trial. Lancet 2009;374:1243-51.

Chaturvedi AK, Caporoso NE, Katki HA, et al. C-reactive protein and risk of lung cancer. J Clin Oncol 2010;28:2719-22.

Gould MK, Maclean CC, Kuscher WG, et al. Accuracy of positron emission tomography for diagnosis of pulmonary nodules and mass lesions: a meta-analysis. JAMA 2001;285:914-24.

Lung. In: Edge SB, Byrd DR, Compton CC, eds. *AJCC Cancer Staging Manual.* 7th ed. New York, NY: Springer, 2010, pp. 253-70.

Fischer B, Lassen U, Mortensen J, et al. Preoperative staging of lung cancer with combined PET-CT. N Eng J Med 2009;361:32-9.

Maziak DE, Darling GE, Inculet RI, et al. Positron emission tomography in staging early lung cancer: a randomized trial. Ann Intern Med 2009;151:221-8.

Herth F, Becker HD, Ernst A. Conventional vs endobronchial ultrasound-guided transbronchial needle aspiration: a randomized trial. Chest 2004;125:322-5.

Arriagada AR, Bergman B, Dunant A, et al. Cisplatin-based adjuvant chemotherapy in patients with completely resected non-small-cell lung cancer. N Eng J med 2004; 350:351-60.

Kato H, Ichinose Y, Ohta M, et al. A randomized trial of adjuvant chemotherapy with uracil-tegafur for adenocarcinoma of the lung. N Eng J Med 2004;350:1713-21.

Winton T, Livingston R, Johnson D, et al. Vinorelbine plus cisplatin vs. observation in resected non-small-cell lung cancer. N Eng J Med 2005;352:2589-97.

NCSLC Meta-analysis Collaborative Group. Adjuvant chemotherapy, with or without postoperative radiotherapy, in operable non-small-cell lung cancer: two meta-analyses of individual patient data. Lancet 2010;375:1267-77.

Trodella L, Granone P, Valente S, et al. Adjuvant radiotherapy in non-small cell lung cancer with pathological stage I: definitive results of a phase III randomized trial. Radiother Oncol 2002;62:11-19.

The Lung Cancer Study Group. Effects of postoperative mediastinal radiation on completely resected stage II and stage III epidermoid cancer of the lung. N Eng J Med 1986;315:1377-81.

PORT Meta-analysis Trialists Group. Postoperative radiotherapy in non-small-cell lung cancer: systematic review and meta-analysis of individual patient data from nine randomized controlled trials. Lancet 1998;352:257-63.

Dillman RO, Seagren SL, Propert KJ, et al. A randomized trial of induction chemotherapy plus high-dose radiation versus radiation alone in stage III non-small-cell lung cancer. N Eng J Med 1990;323:940-5.

Sause W, Kolesar P, Taylor S, et al. Final results of a phase III trial in regionally unresectable non-small cell lung cancer: Radiation Therapy Oncology Group, Eastern Cooperative Oncology Group, and Southwest Oncology Group. Chest 2000;117:358-64.

Schaake-Koning C, van den Bogaert W, et al. Effects of concomitant cisplatin and radiotherapy on inoperable non-small cell lung cancer. N Eng J Med 1992;326:524-30.

Jeremic B, Shibamoto Y, Acimovic L, Djuric L. Randomized trial of hyperfractionated radiation therapy with or without concurrent chemotherapy for stage III non-small-cell lung cancer. J Clin Oncol 1995;13:452-8.

Furuse K, Fukuoka M, Kawahara M, et al. Phase III study of concurrent versus sequential thoracic radiotherapy in combination with mitomycin, vindesine, and cisplatin in unresectable stage III non-small-cell lung cancer. J Clin Oncol 1999;17:2692-9.

Albain KS, Swann RS, Rusch VW, et al. Radiotherapy plus chemotherapy with or without surgical resection for stage III non-small cell lung cancer: a phase III randomized controlled trial. Lancet 2009;374:379-386.

Auperin A, LePechoux C, Rolland E, et al. Meta-analysis of concomitant versus sequential radiochemotherapy in locally advanced non-small-cell lung cancer. J Clin Oncol 2010;28:2181-90.

Schiller JH, Harrington D, Belani CP, et al. Comparison of four chemotherapy regimens for advanced non-small-cell lung cancer. N Eng J Med 2002;346:92-8.

Sandler A, Gray R, Perry MC, et al. Paclitaxel-carboplatin alone or with bevacizumab for non-small-cell lung cancer. N Eng J Med 2006;355:2542-50.

Maemondo M, Inoue A, Kobayashi K, et al. Gefitinib or chemotherapy for non-small-cell lung cancer with mutated EGFR. N Eng J Med 2010;362:2380-8.

Kim ES, Hirsh V, Mok T, et al. Gefitinib versus docetaxel in previously treated non-small-cell lung cancer (INTEREST): a randomized trial. Lancet 2008;372:1809-18.

Shepherd FA, Rodrigues Pereira J, Ciuleanu T, et al. Erlotinib in previously treated non-small-cell lung cancer. N Eng J Med 2005;353:123-32.

Perry MC, Eaton WL, Propert KJ, et al. Chemotherapy with or without radiation therapy in limited stage small-cell lung cancer. N Eng J Med 1987;316:912-8.

Turrisi AT, Kim K, Blum R, et al. Twice-daily compared with once-daily thoracic radiotherapy in limited small-cell lung cancer treated concurrently with cisplatin and etoposide. N Eng J Med 1999;340:265-71.

Auperin A, Arriagada R, Pignon JP, et al. Prophylactic cranial irradiation for patients with small-cell lung cancer in complete remission. Prophylactic Cranial Irradiation Overview Collaborative Group. N Eng J Med 1999;341:476-84.

Slotman B, Faivre-Finn C, Kramer G, et al. Prophylactic cranial irradiation in extensive small-cell lung cancer. N Eng J med 2007;357:664-72.

LYMPHOMA, NON-HODGKIN

Altekruse SF, Kosary CL, Krapcho M, Neyman N, Aminou R, Waldron W, Ruhl J, Howlader N, Tatalovich Z, Cho H, Mariotto A, Eisner MP, Lewis DR, Cronin K, Chen HS, Feuer EJ, Stinchcomb DG, Edwards BK (eds). SEER Cancer Statistics Review, 1975-2007, National Cancer Institute. Bethesda, MD, http://seer.cancer.gov/csr/1975_2007/, based on November 2009 SEER data submission, posted to the SEER web site, 2010.

Parsonnet J, Isaacson PG. Bacterial infection and MALT lymphoma. N Eng J Med 2004;350:213-5.

Chen LT, Lin JT, Tai JJ, et al. Long-term results of anti-helicobacter pylori therapy in early-stage gastric high-grade transformed MALT lymphoma. J Natl Cancer Inst 2005;97:1345-53.

Hodgkin and Non-Hodgkin Lymphomas. In: Edge SB, Byrd DR, Compton CC, eds. *AJCC Cancer Staging Manual.* 7th ed. New York, NY: Springer, 2010, pp. 607-16.

Ansell SM, Armitage J. Non-Hodgkin lymphoma: diagnosis and treatment. Mayo Clin Proc 2005;80:1087-97.

Jerusalem G, Beguin Y, Fassotte MF, et al. Whole-body positron emission tomography using 18F-fluorodeoxyglucose for posttreatment evaluation in Hodgkin's disease and non-Hodgkin's lymphoma has higher diagnostic and prognostic value than classical computed tomography scan imaging. Blood 1999;94:429-33.

Kwee TC, Kwee RM, Nievelstein RA. Imaging in staging of malignant lymphoma: a systematic review. Blood 2008;111:504-16.

Ziepert M, Hasenclever D, Kuhnt E, et al. Standard International Prognostic Index remains a valid predictor of outcome for patients with aggressive CD20+ B-cell lymphoma in the rituximab era. J Clin Oncol 2010;28:2373-6.

Slal-Celigny P, Roy P, Colombat P, et al. Follicular lymphoma international prognostic index. Blood 2004;104:1258-65.

Fisher RI, Gaynor ER, Dahlberg S, et al. Comparison of a standard regimen (CHOP) with three intensive chemotherapy regimens for advanced non-Hodgkin's lymphoma. N Eng J Med 1993;328:1002-6.

Tirelli U, Errante D, Van Glabbeke M, et al. CHOP is the standard regimen in patients > or = 70 years of age with intermediate-grade and high-grade non-Hodgkin's lymphoma: results of a randomized study of the European Organization for research and Treatment of Cancer Lymphoma Cooperative Study Group. J Clin Oncol 1998;16:27-34.

Miller TP, Dahlberg S, Cassady JR, et al. Chemotherapy alone compared with chemotherapy plus radiotherapy for localized intermediate- and high-grade non-Hodgkin's lymphoma. N Eng J Med 1998;339:21-6.

Schlembach PJ, Wilder RB, Tucker SL, et al. Impact of involved field radiotherapy after CHOP-based chemotherapy on stage III-IV, intermediate grade and large-cell immunoblastic lymphomas. Int J Radiat Oncol Biol Phys 2000;48:1107-10.

Haioun C, Lepage E, Gisselbrecht C, et al. Comparison of autologous bone marrow transplantation with sequential chemotherapy for intermediate-grade and high-grade non-Hodgkin's lymphoma in first complete remission: a study of 464 patients. Group d'Etude des Lymphomes de l'Adulte. J Clin Oncol 1994;12:2543-51.

Haioun C, Lepage E, Gisselbrecht C, et al. Survival benefit of high-dose therapy in poor-risk aggressive non-Hodgkin's lymphoma: final analysis of the prospective LNH87-2 protocol—a groupe d'Etud des lymphomes de l'Adulte study. J Clin Oncol 2000; 18:3025-30.

Hagenbeek A, Eghbali H, Monfardini S, et al. Phase III intergroup study of fludarabine phosphate compared with cyclophosphamide, vincristine, and prednisone chemotherapy in newly diagnosed patients with stage III and IV low-grade malignant Non-Hodgkin's lymphoma. J Clin Oncol 2006;24:1590-6.

Tsang RW, Gospodarowicz MK. Radiation therapy for localized low-grade non-Hodgkin's lymphomas. Hematol Oncol 2005;23:10-7.

MacManus MP, Hoppe RT. Is radiotherapy curative for stage I and II low-grade follicular lymphoma? Results of a long-term follow-up study of patients treated at Stanford University. J Clin Oncol 1996;14:1282-90.

Bartlett NL, Rizeq M, Dorfman RF, et al. Follicular large-cell lymphoma: intermediate or low grade? J Clin Oncol 1994;12:1349-57.

MELANOMA

Altekruse SF, Kosary CL, Krapcho M, Neyman N, Aminou R, Waldron W, Ruhl J, Howlader N, Tatalovich Z, Cho H, Mariotto A, Eisner MP, Lewis DR, Cronin K, Chen HS, Feuer EJ, Stinchcomb DG, Edwards BK (eds). SEER Cancer Statistics Review, 1975-2007, National Cancer Institute. Bethesda, MD, http://seer.cancer.gov/csr/1975_2007/, based on November 2009 SEER data submission, posted to the SEER web site, 2010

Rhodes AR, Weinstock MA, Fitzpatrick TB, et al. Risk factors for cutaneous melanoma. A practical method of recognizing predisposed individuals. JAMA 1987;258:3146-54.

Rager EL, Bridgeford EP, Ollila DW. Cutaneous melanoma: update on prevention, screening, diagnosis, and treatment. Am Fam Physician 2005;72:269-76.

Tsao H, Bevona C, Goggins W, Quinn T. The transformation rate of moles (melanocytic nevi) into cutaneous melanoma: a population-based estimate. Arch Dermatol 2003;139:282-8.

Finck SJ, Giuliano AE, Morton DL. LDH and melanoma. Cancer 1983;51:840-3.

Balch CM, Soong SJ, Atkins MB, et al. An evidence-based staging system for cutaneous melanoma. CA Cancer J Clin 2004;54:131-49.

Melanoma of the Skin. In: Edge SB, Byrd DR, Compton CC, eds. *AJCC Cancer Staging Manual.* 7th ed. New York, NY: Springer, 2010, pp. 325-44.

Morton DL, Thompson JF, Cochran AJ, et al. Sentinel-node biopsy or nodal observation in melanoma. N Eng J Med 2006;355:1307-17.

Grob JJ, Dreno B, de la Salmoniere P, et al. Randomized trial of interferon alpha-2a as adjuvant therapy in resected primary melanoma thicker than 1.5 mm without clinically detectable node metastases. French Cooperative Group on Melanoma. Lancet 1998;351:1905-10.

Eggermont AM, Suciu S, MacKie R, et al. Post-surgery adjuvant therapy with intermediate doses of interferon alfa 2b versus observation in patients with stage IIb/III melanoma (EORTC 18952): randomized controlled trial. Lancet 2005;366:1189-96.

Cascinelli N, Belli F, MacKie RM, et al. Effect of long-term adjuvant therapy with interferon alpha-2a in patients with regional node metastases from cutaneous melanoma: a randomized trial. Lancet 2001;358:866-9.

Eggermont AM, Suciu S, Santinami M, et al. Adjuvant therapy with pegylated interferon alfa-2b versus observation alone in resected stage III melanoma: final results of EORTC 18991, a randomized phase III trial. Lancet 2008;372:117-26.

Bottomley A, Coens C, Suciu S, et al. Adjuvant therapy with pegylated interferon alfa-2b versus observation in resected stage III melanoma: a phase III randomized controlled trial of health-related quality of life and symptoms by the European Organization for Research and Treatment of Cancer Melanoma Group. J Clin Oncol 2009;27:2916-23.

Mocellin S, Pasquali S, Rossi CR, Nitti D. Interferon alpha adjuvant therapy in patients with high-risk melanoma: a systematic review and meta-analysis. J Natl Cancer Inst 2010;102:493-501.

Eton O Legha SS, Bedikian AY, et al. Sequential biochemotherapy versus chemotherapy for metastatic melanoma: results from a phase III randomized trial. J Clin Oncol 2002;20:2045-52.

Atkins MB, Hsu J, Lee S, et al. Phase III trial comparing concurrent biochemotherapy with cisplatin, vinblastine, and dacarbazine alone in patients with metastatic melanoma (E3695): a trial coordinated by the Easter Cooperative Oncology Group. J Clin Oncol 2008;26:5748-54.

Hodi FS, O'Day SJ, McDermott DF, et al. Improved survival with ipilimumab in patients with metastatic melanoma. N Eng J Med 2010;363:711-23.

MYELOMA

Altekruse SF, Kosary CL, Krapcho M, Neyman N, Aminou R, Waldron W, Ruhl J, Howlader N, Tatalovich Z, Cho H, Mariotto A, Eisner MP, Lewis DR, Cronin K, Chen HS, Feuer EJ, Stinchcomb DG, Edwards BK (eds). SEER Cancer Statistics Review, 1975-2007, National Cancer Institute. Bethesda, MD, http://seer.cancer.gov/csr/1975_2007/, based on November 2009 SEER data submission, posted to the SEER web site, 2010.

Ludwig H, Durie BG, Bolejack V, et al. Myeloma in patients younger than age 50 years presents with more favorable features and shows better survival: an analysis of 10,549 patients from the International Myeloma Working Group. Blood 2008;111:4039-47.

Kyle RA. Monoclonal gammopathy of undetermined significance. Blood Rev 1994;8:135-41.

Multiple Myeloma and Plasma Cell Disorders. In: Edge SB, Byrd DR, Compton CC, eds. *AJCC Cancer Staging Manual.* 7th ed. New York, NY: Springer, 2010, pp. 617-18.

Lahtinen R, Laakso M, Palva I, et al. Randomized, placebo-controlled multicentre trial of clodronate in multiple myeloma. Finnish Leukaemia Group. Lancet 1992;340:1049-52.

Behrenson JR, Lichtenstein A, Porter L, et al. Efficacy of pamidronate in reducing skeletal events in patients with advanced multiple myeloma. Myeloma Aredia Study Group. N Eng J med 1996;334:488-93.

Attal M, Harousseau JL, Stoppa AM, et al. A prospective, randomized trial of autologous bone marrow transplantation and chemotherapy in multiple myeloma. Intergroupe Francais du Myelome. N Eng J med 1996;335:91-7.

Child JA, Morgan GJ, Davies FE, et al. High-dose chemotherapy with hematopoietic stem-cell rescue for multiple myeloma. N Eng J Med 2003;348:1875-83.

Fermand JP, Katsahian S, Divine M, et al. High-dose therapy and autologous blood stem-cell transplantation compared with conventional treatment in myeloma patients aged 55 to 65 years: long-term results of a randomized control trial from the Group Myelome-Autogreffe. J Clin Oncol 2005;23:9227-33.

Barlogie B, Tricot G, Aniaaie E, et al. Thalidomide and hematopoietic-cell transplantation for multiple myeloma. N Eng J Med 2006;354:1021-30.

Rotta M, Storer BE, Sahabi F, et al. Long-term outcome of patients with multiple myeloma after autologous hematopoietic cell transplantation and nonmyeloablative allografting. Blood 2009;113:3383-91.

Lokhorst HM, van der Holt B, Zweegman S, et al. A randomized phase 3 study on the effect of thalidomide combined with adriamycin, dexamethasone, and high-dose melphalan, followed by thalidomide maintenance in patients with multiple myeloma. Blood 2010;115:1113-20.

Facon T, Mary JY, Hulin C, et al. Melphelan and prednisone plus thalidomide versus melphalan and prednisone alone or reduced-intensity autologous stem cell transplantation in elderly patients with multiple myeloma (IFM 99-06): a randomized trial. Lancet 2007;370:1209-18.

Palumbo A, Bringhen S, Liberati AM, et al. Oral melphalan, prednisone, and thalidomide in elderly patients with multiple myeloma: updated results of a randomized controlled trial. Blood 2008;112:3107-14.

Hulin C, Facon T, Rodon P, et al. Efficacy of melphalan and prednisone plus thalidomide in patients older than 75 years with newly diagnosed multiple myeloma: IFM 01/01 trial. J Clin Oncol 2009;27:3664-70.

Mateos MV, Richardson PG, Schlag R, et al. Bortezomib plus melphalan and prednisone compared with mephalan and prednisone in previously untreated multiple myeloma: updated follow-up and impact of subsequent therapy in the phase III VISTA trial. J Clin Oncol 2010;28:2259-66.

Dimopoulos M, Spencer A, Attal M, et al. Lenalidomide plus dexamethasone for relapsed or refractory multiple myeloma. N Eng J Med 2007;357:2123-32.

Weber DM, Chen C, Niesvizky R, et al. Lenalidomide plus dexamethasone for relapsed multiple myeloma in North America. N Eng J Med 2007;357:2133-42.

OVARIAN CANCER

Altekruse SF, Kosary CL, Krapcho M, Neyman N, Aminou R, Waldron W, Ruhl J, Howlader N, Tatalovich Z, Cho H, Mariotto A, Eisner MP, Lewis DR, Cronin K, Chen HS, Feuer EJ, Stinchcomb DG, Edwards BK (eds). SEER Cancer Statistics Review, 1975-2007, National Cancer Institute. Bethesda, MD, http://seer.cancer.gov/csr/1975_2007/, based on November 2009 SEER data submission, posted to the SEER web site, 2010.

Makar AP, Kristensen GB, Kaern J, et al. Prognostic value of pre- and postoperative serum CA 125 levels in ovarian cancer: new aspects and multivariate analysis. Obstet Gynecol 1992;79:1002-10.

Paramasivam S, Tripcony L, Crandon A, et al. Prognostic importance of preoperative CA-125 in International Federation of Gynecology and Obstetrics stage I epithelial ovarian cancer: an Australian multicenter study. J Clin Oncol 2005;23:5938-42.

Ovary and Primary Peritoneal Carcinoma. In: Edge SB, Byrd DR, Compton CC, eds. *AJCC Cancer Staging Manual.* 7th ed. New York, NY: Springer, 2010, pp. 419-28.

Baker TR, Piver MS, Hempling RE. Long-term survival by cytoreductive surgery to less than 1cm, induction weekly cisplatin and monthly cisplatin, doxorubicin, and cyclophosphamide in advanced ovarian adenocarcinoma. Cancer 1994;74:656-63.

Wimberger P, Lehmann N, Kimmig R, et al. Prognostic factors for complete debulking in advanced ovarian cancer and its impact on survival. An exploratory analysis of a prospectively randomized phase III study of the Arbeitsgemeinschaft Gynaekologische Onkologie Ovarian Cancer Study Group (AGO-OVAR). Gynecol Oncol 2007;106:69-74.

Rose PG, Nerenstone S, Brady MF, et al. Secondary surgical cytoreduction for advanced ovarian carcinoma. N Eng J Med 2004;351:2489-97.

McGuire WP, Hoskins WJ, Brady MF, et al. Cyclophosphamide and cisplatin compared with paclitaxel and cisplatin in patients with stage III and stage IV ovarian cancer. N Eng J Med 1996;334:1-6.

Piccart NM, Bettelson K, James K, et al. Randomized intergroup trial of cisplatin-paclitaxel versus cisplatin cyclophosphamide in women with advanced epithelial ovarian cancer: three year results. J Natl Cancer Inst 2000;92: 699-708.

Ozols RF, Bundy BN, Greer E, et al. Phase III trials of carboplatin and paclitaxel compared with cisplatin and paclitaxel in patients with optimally resected stage III ovarian cancer: a Gynecologic Oncology Group Study. J Clin Oncol 2003;21:3194-3200.

International Collaborative Ovarian Neoplasm Group Paclitaxel plus carboplatin versus standard chemotherapy with either single agent carboplatin or cyclophosphamide, doxorubicin, and cisplatin in women with ovarian cancer: the ICON3 randomized trial. Lancet 2002;360:505-15.

Alberts DS, Liu PY. Hannigan EV, et al. Intraperitoneal cisplatin plus intravenous cyclophosphamide versus intravenous cisplatin plus intravenous cyclophosphamide for stage III ovarian cancer. N Eng J Med 1996;335:1950-5.

Armstrong DK, Bundy B, Wenzel L, et al. Intraperitoneal cisplatin and paclitaxel in ovarian cancer. N Eng J Med 2006;354:34-43.

Dembo AJ. Abdominopelvic radiotherapy in ovarian cancer. A 10-year experience. Cancer 1985;55:2285-90.

PANCREATIC CANCER

Altekruse SF, Kosary CL, Krapcho M, Neyman N, Aminou R, Waldron W, Ruhl J, Howlader N, Tatalovich Z, Cho H, Mariotto A, Eisner MP, Lewis DR, Cronin K, Chen HS, Feuer EJ, Stinchcomb DG, Edwards BK (eds). SEER Cancer Statistics Review, 1975-2007, National Cancer Institute. Bethesda, MD, http://seer.cancer.gov/csr/1975_2007/, based on November 2009 SEER data submission, posted to the SEER web site, 2010

Exocrine and Endocrine Pancreas. In: Edge SB, Byrd DR, Compton CC, eds. *AJCC Cancer Staging Manual.* 7th ed. New York, NY: Springer, 2010, pp. 241-50.

Pedrazzoli S, DiCarlo V, Dionigi R, et al. Standard versus extended lymphadenectomy associated with pancreaticoduodenectomy in the surgical treatment of adenocarcinoma of the head of the pancreas: a multicenter, prospective, randomized study. Lymphadenectomy Study Group. Ann Surg 1998;228:508-17.

Farnell MB, Pearson RK, Sarr MG, et al. A prospective randomized trial comparing standard pancreaticoduodenectomy with pancreaticoduodenectomy with extended lymphadenectomy in resectable pancreatic head adenocarcinoma. Surgery 2005;138:618-28.

Kalser M, Ellenberg S. Pancreatic Cancer. Adjuvant combined radiation and chemotherapy following curative resection. Arch Surg 1985;120:899-903.GITSG 91-73

Neoptolemos JP, Stocken DD, Friess H, et al. A randomized trial of chemoradiotherapy and chemotherapy after resection of pancreatic cancer. N Eng J Med 2004;350:1200-10.

Klinkenbijl JH, Jeekel J, Sahmoud T, et al. Adjuvant radiotherapy and 5-fluorouracil after curative resection of cancer of the pancreas and periampullary region: phase III trial of the EORTC gastrointestinal tract cancer cooperative group. Ann Surg 1999;230:776-82.

Smeenk HG, van Eijck CH, Hop WC, et al. Long-term survival and metastatic pattern of pancreatic and periampullary cancer after adjuvant chemoradiation or observation: long-term results of EORTC trial 40891. Ann Surg 2007;246:734-40.

Oettle H, Post S, Neuhaus P, et al. Adjuvant chemotherapy with gemcitabine vs observation in patients undergoing curative-intent resection of pancreatic cancer: a randomized controlled trial. JAMA 2007;297:267-77.

Regine WF, Winter KA, Abrams RA, et al. Fluorouracil vs gemcitabine chemotherapy before and after fluorouracil-based chemoradiation following resection of pancreatic adenocarcinoma: a randomized controlled trial. JAMA 2008;299:1019-26.

Moertel CG, Frytak S, Hahn RG, et al. Therapy of locally unresectable pancreatic carcinoma: a randomized comparison of high dose (6000 rads) radiation alone, moderate dose radiation (4000 rads + 5-fluorouracil), and high dose radiation + 5-fluorouracil: The Gastrointestinal Tumor Study Group. Cancer 1981;48:1705-10.

PROSTATE CANCER

Altekruse SF, Kosary CL, Krapcho M, Neyman N, Aminou R, Waldron W, Ruhl J, Howlader N, Tatalovich Z, Cho H, Mariotto A, Eisner MP, Lewis DR, Cronin K, Chen HS, Feuer EJ, Stinchcomb DG, Edwards BK (eds). SEER Cancer Statistics Review, 1975-2007, National Cancer Institute. Bethesda, MD, http://seer.cancer.gov/csr/1975_2007/, based on November 2009 SEER data submission, posted to the SEER web site, 2010

Prostate. In: Edge SB, Byrd DR, Compton CC, eds. *AJCC Cancer Staging Manual.* 7th ed. New York, NY: Springer, 2010, pp. 457-68.

Partin AW, Kattan MW, Subong EN, et al. Combination of prostate-specific antigen, clinical stage, and Gleason score to predict pathological stage of localized prostate cancer: a multi-institutional update. JAMA 1997;277:1445-51.

D'Amico AV, Cote K, Loffredo M, et al. Determinants of prostate cancer-specific survival after radiation therapy for patients with clinically localized prostate cancer. J Clin Oncol 2002;20:4567-73.

Sebo TJ, Bock BJ, Cheville JC, et al. The percent of cores positive for cancer in prostate needle biopsy specimens is strongly predictive of tumor stage and volume at radical prostatectomy. J Urol 2000;163:174-8.

Chodak GW, Thisted RA, Gerber GS, et al. Results of conservative management of clinically localized prostate cancer. N Eng J Med 1994;330:242-8.

Albertson PC, Fryback DG, Storer BE, et al. Long-term survival among men with conservatively treated localized prostate cancer. JAMA 1995;274:626-31.

Johannson JE, Andren O, Andersson SO, et al. Natural history of early, localized prostate cancer. JAMA 2004;291:2713-19.

Han M, Partin AW, Pound CR, et al. Long-term biochemical disease-free and cancer-specific survival following anatomic radical retropubic prostatectomy. The 15-year Johns Hopkins Experience. Urol Clin North Am 2001;28:555-65.

Fowler FJ, Roman A, Barry MJ, et al. Patient-reported complications and follow-up treatment after radical prostatectomy, the national Medicare experience: 1988-1990 (updated June 1993). Urol 1993;42:622-29.

Stanford JL, Feng Z, Hamilton AS, et al. Urinary and sexual function after radical prostatectomy for clinically localized prostate cancer: The Prostate Cancer Outcomes Study. JAMA 2000;283:354-60.

Lasser MS, Renzulli J, Turini GA, et al. An unbiased prospective report of perioperative complications of robot-assisted laparoscopic radical prostatectomy. Urol 2010; 75:1083-9.

Nelson B, Kaufman M, Broughton G, et al. Comparison of length of hospital stay between retropubic prostatectomy and robotic laparoscopic assisted prostatectomy. J Urol 2007;177:929-31.

Barocas DA, Salem S, Kordan Y, et al. Robotic assisted laparoscopic prostatectomy versus radical retropubic prostatectomy for clinically localized prostate cancer: comparison of short-term biochemical recurrence-free survival. J Urol 2010;183:990-6.

D'Amico AV, Whittington R, Malkowicz B, et al. Biochemical outcome after radical prostatectomy, external beam radiation therapy, or interstitial radiation therapy for clinically localized prostate cancer. JAMA 1998;280:969-74.

Beyer DC, Thomas T, Hilbe J, et al. Relative influence of Gleason score and pretreatment PSA in predicting survival following brachytherapy for prostate cancer. Brachytherapy 2003;2:77-84.

Potters L, Morganstern C, Calugaru E, et al. 12-year outcomes following permanent prostate brachytherapy for patients with clinically localized prostate cancer. J Urol 2005;173:1562-6.

Hinnen KA, Batterman JJ, van Roermund JG, et al. Long-term biochemical and survival outcome of 921 patients treated with I-125 permanent prostate brachytherapy. In t J Radiat Oncol Biol Phys 2010;76:1433-8.

Zeitman AL, Bae K, Slater JD, et al. Randomized trial comparing conventional-dose with high-dose conformal radiation therapy in early-stage adenocarcinoma of the prostate: long-term results from proton radiation oncology group/American college of radiology 95-09. J Clin Oncol 2010;28:1106-11.

Fowler FF, Barry MJ, Lu-Yao GL, et al. Outcomes of external-beam radiation therapy for prostate cancer: a study of Medicare beneficiaries in three surveillance, epidemiology, and end results areas. J Clin Oncol 1996;14:2258-65.

Sanda MG, Dunn RL, Michalski J, et al., Quality of life and Satisfaction with Outcome among Prostate Cancer Survivors. N Eng J Med 2008;358:1250-61.

D'Amico AV, Manola J, Loffredo M, et al. 6-month androgen suppression plus radiation therapy vs radiation therapy alone for patients with clinically localized prostate cancer: a randomized controlled trial. JAMA 2004;292:821-7.

Bolla M, Gonzalez D, Warde P, et al. Improved survival in patients with locally advanced prostate cancer treated with radiotherapy and goserelin. N Eng J Med 1997;337:295-300.

Pilepich MV, Winter K, John MJ, et al. Phase III radiation therapy oncology group (RTOG) trial 86-10 of androgen deprivation adjuvant to definitive radiotherapy in locally advanced carcinoma of the prostate. Int J Radiat Oncol Biol Phys 2001;50:1243-52.

Denham JW, Steigler A, Lamb DS, et al. Short-term androgen deprivation and radiotherapy for locally advanced prostate cancer: results from the Trans-Tasman Radiation Oncology Group 96.01 randomized controlled trial. Lancet Oncol 2005;6:841-50.

D'Amico AV, Moran BJ, Braccioforte MH, et al. Risk of death from prostate cancer after brachytherapy alone or with radiation, androgen suppression therapy, or both in men with high-risk disease. J Clin Oncol 2009;27:3923-8.

Prostate Cancer Trialists' Collaborative Group. Maximum androgen blockade in advanced prostate cancer: an overview of randomized trials. Lancet 2000;355:1491-8.

Widmark A, Klepp O, Solberg A, et al. Endocrine treatment, with or without radiotherapy, in locally advanced prostate cancer (SPCG-7/SFUO-3): an open randomized phase III trial. Lancet 2009;373:301-8.

Pound CR, Partin AW, Eisenberger MA, et al. Natural history of progression after PSA elevation following radical prostatectomy. JAMA 1999;281:1591-7.

Bolla M, van Poppel H, Collette L, et al. Postoperative radiotherapy after radical prostatectomy: a randomized controlled trial (EORTC 22911). Lancet 2005;366:572-8.

Wiegel T, Bottke D, Steiner U, et el. Phase III postoperative adjuvant radiotherapy after radical prostatectomy compared with radical prostatectomy alone in pT3 prostate cancer with postoperative undetectable prostate-specific antigen: ARO 96-02/AUO 09/95.

Thompson IM, Tangen CM, Paradelo J, et al. Adjuvant radiotherapy for pathological T3N0M0 prostate cancer significantly reduces risk of metastases and improves survival: long-term followup of a randomized clinical trial. J Urol 2009;181:956-62.

Van Cangh PJ, Richard F, Lorge F, et al. Adjuvant radiation therapy does not cause urinary incontinence after radical prostatectomy: results of a prospective randomized study. J Urol 1998;159:164-6.

Bastasch MD, The BS, Mai WY, et al. Post-nerve-sparing prostatectomy, dose-escalated intensity-modulated radiotherapy: effect on erectile function. Int J Radiat Oncol Biol Phys 2002;54:101-6.

Kantoff PW, Higano CS, Shore ND, et al. Sipuleucel-T immunotherapy for castration-resistant prostate cancer. N Eng J Med 2010;363:411-22.

SKIN CANCER, NONMELANOMA

Altekruse SF, Kosary CL, Krapcho M, Neyman N, Aminou R, Waldron W, Ruhl J, Howlader N, Tatalovich Z, Cho H, Mariotto A, Eisner MP, Lewis DR, Cronin K, Chen HS, Feuer EJ, Stinchcomb DG, Edwards BK (eds). SEER Cancer Statistics Review, 1975-2007, National Cancer Institute. Bethesda, MD, http://seer.cancer.gov/csr/1975_2007/, based on November 2009 SEER data submission, posted to the SEER web site, 2010.

Karagas MR, Stukel TA, Greenberg ER, et al. Risk of subsequent basal cell carcinoma and squamous cell carcinoma of the skin among patients with prior skin cancer. Skin Cancer Prevention Study Group. JAMA 1992;267:3305-10.

Thompson SC, Jolley D, Marks R. Reduction of solar keratoses by regular sunscreen use. N Eng J Med 1993;329:1147-51.

Black HS, Herd JA, Goldberg LH, et al. Effect of a low-fat diet on the incidence of actinic keratosis. N Eng J Med 1994;330:1272-5.

Karagas MR, MacDonald JA, Greenberg ER, et al. Risk of basal cell and squamous cell skin cancers after ionizing radiation therapy. For The Skin Cancer Prevention Study Group. J Natl Cancer Inst 1996;88:1848-53.

Green A, Williams G, Neale R, et al. Daily sunscreen application and beta-carotene supplementation in prevention of basal-cell and squamous-cell carcinomas of the skin: a randomized controlled trial. Lancet 1999;354:723-9.

Cutaneous Squamous Cell Carcinoma and Other Cutaneous Carcinomas. In: Edge SB, Byrd DR, Compton CC, eds. *AJCC Cancer Staging Manual.* 7th ed. New York, NY: Springer, 2010, pp. 301-14.

Morton C, Horn M, Leman J, et al. Comparison of topical methyl aminolevulinate photodynamic therapy with cryotherapy or fluorouracil for treatment of squamous cell carcinoma in situ: results of a multicenter randomized trial. Arch Dermatol 2006;142:729-35.

Rhodes LE, de Rie MA, Leifsdottir R, et al. Five-year follow-up of a randomized, prospective trial of topical methyl aminolevulinate photodynamic therapy vs surgery for nodular basal cell carcinoma. Arch Dermatol 2007;143:1131-6.

Roenig RK. Mohs' micrographic surgery. Mayo Clin Proc 1988;63:175-83.

Mosterd K, Krekels GA, Nieman FH, et al. Surgical excision versus Mohs' micrographic surgery for primary and recurrent basal-cell carcinoma of the face: a prospective randomized controlled trial with 5-years' follow-up. Lancet Oncol 2008;9:1149-56.

Petrovich Z, Kuisk H, Langholz B, et al. Treatment results and patterns of failure in 646 patients with carcinoma of the eyelids, pinna, and nose. Am J Surg 1987;154:447-50.

Mazeron JJ, Chassagne D, Crook J, et al. Radiation therapy of carcinomas of the skin of nose and nasal vestibule: a report of 1646 cases by the Groupe Europeen de Curietherape. Radiother Oncol 1988;13:165-73.

Mendenhall WM, Amdur RJ, Hinerman RW, et al. Radiotherapy for cutaneous squamous cell and basal cell carcinomas of the head and neck. Laryngoscope 2009;119:1994-9.

Lovett RD, Perez CA, Shapiro SJ, Garcia DM. External irradiation of epithelial skin cancer. Int J Radiat Oncol Biol Phys 1990;19:235-42.

Petiti JY, Avril MF, Margulis A, et al. Evaluation of cosmetic results of a randomized trial comparing surgery and radiotherapy in the treatment of basal cell carcinoma of the face. Plast Reconstr Surg 2000;105:2544-51.

Bernier J, Domenge C, Ozsahin M, et al. Postoperative irradiation with or without concomitant chemotherapy for locally advanced head and neck cancer. N Eng J Med 2004;350:1945-52.

Cooper JS, Pajak TF, Forastiere AA, et al. Postoperative concurrent radiotherapy and chemotherapy for high-risk squamous-cell carcinoma of the head and neck. N Eng J Med 2004;350:1937-44.

STOMACH CANCER

Altekruse SF, Kosary CL, Krapcho M, Neyman N, Aminou R, Waldron W, Ruhl J, Howlader N, Tatalovich Z, Cho H, Mariotto A, Eisner MP, Lewis DR, Cronin K, Chen HS, Feuer EJ, Stinchcomb DG, Edwards BK (eds). SEER Cancer Statistics Review, 1975-2007, National Cancer Institute. Bethesda, MD, http://seer.cancer.gov/csr/1975_2007/, based on November 2009 SEER data submission, posted to the SEER web site, 2010

Fuccio L, Zagari RM, Eusebi LH, et al. Meta-analysis: can Helicobacter pylori eradication treatment reduce the risk for gastric cancer? Ann Intern Med 2009;151:121-8.

Horie Y, Niura K, Matsui K, et al. Marked elevation of plasma carcinoembryonic antigen and stomach carcinoma. Cancer 1996;77:1991-7.

Stomach. In: Edge SB, Byrd DR, Compton CC, eds. *AJCC Cancer Staging Manual.* 7th ed. New York, NY: Springer, 2010, pp. 117-26.

Bozzetti F, Marubini E, Bonfanti G, et al. Subtotal versus total gastrectomy for gastric cancer: five-year survival rates in a multicenter randomized Italian trial. Italian Gastrointestinal Tumor Study Group. Ann Surg 1999;230:170-8.

Huscher CG, Mingoli A, Sgarzini G, et al. Laparoscopic versus open subtotal gastrectomy for distal gastric cancer: five-year results of a randomized prospective trial. Ann Surg 2005;241:232-7.

Strong VE, Devaud N, Allen PJ, et al. Laparoscopic versus open subtotal gastrectomy for adenocarcinoma: a case-control study. Ann Surg Oncol 2009;16:1507-13.

Kim YW, Baik YH, Yun YH, et al. Improved quality of life outcomes after laparoscopy-assisted distal gastrectomy for early gastric cancer: results of a prospective randomized clinical trial. Ann Surg 2008;248:721-7.

Sasako M, Sano T, Yamamoto S, et al. D2 lymphadenectomy alone or with para-aortic nodal dissection for gastric cancer. N Eng J Med 2008;359:453-62.

Songun I, Putter H, Kranenbarg EM, et al. Surgical treatment of gastric cancer: 15-year follow-up results of the randomized nationwide Dutch D1D2 trial. Lancet Oncol 2010;11:439-49.

MacDonald JS, Smalley SR, Benedetti J et al. Chemoradiotherapy after surgery compared with surgery alone for adenocarcinoma of the stomach or gastroesophageal junction. N Eng J Med 2001;345:725-30.

Cunningham D, Allum WH, Stenning SP, et al. Perioperative chemotherapy versus surgery alone for resectable gastroesophageal cancer. N Eng J Med 2006;355:11-20.

Dikken JL, Jansen PM, Cats A, et al. Impact of extent of surgery and postoperative chemoradiotherapy on recurrence patterns in gastric cancer. J Clin Oncol 2010;28:2430-6.

Sakuramoto S, Sasako M, Yamaguchi T, et al. Adjuvant chemotherapy for gastric cancer with S-1, an oral fluoropyrimidine. N Eng J Med 2007;357:1810-20.

Koizumi W, Narahara H, Hara T, et al. S-1 plus cisplatin versus S-1 alone for first line treatment of advanced gastric cancer (SPIRITS) trial: a phase III trial. Lancet Oncol 2008;9:215-21.

Cunningham D, Starling N, Rao S, et al. Capecitabine and oxaliplatin for advanced esophagogastric cancer. N Eng J Med 2008;358:36-46.

THYROID CANCER

Altekruse SF, Kosary CL, Krapcho M, Neyman N, Aminou R, Waldron W, Ruhl J, Howlader N, Tatalovich Z, Cho H, Mariotto A, Eisner MP, Lewis DR, Cronin K, Chen HS, Feuer EJ, Stinchcomb DG, Edwards BK (eds). SEER Cancer Statistics Review, 1975-2007, National Cancer Institute. Bethesda, MD, http://seer.cancer.gov/csr/1975_2007/, based on November 2009 SEER data submission, posted to the SEER web site, 2010

De Vathaire F, Hardiman C, Shamsaldin A, et al. Thyroid carcinomas after irradiation for a first cancer during childhood. Arch Intern Med 1999;159:2713-9.

Thyroid. In: Edge SB, Byrd DR, Compton CC, eds. *AJCC Cancer Staging Manual.* 7th ed. New York, NY: Springer, 2010, pp. 87-96.

Holzer S, Reiers C, Mann K, et al. Patterns of care for patients with primary differentiated thyroid carcinoma of the thyroid gland treated in Germany during 1996. U.S. and German Thyroid Cancer Group. Cancer 2000;89:192-201.

Hoang JK, Lee WK, Lee M, et al. US features of thyroid malignancy: pearls and pitfalls. Radiographics 2007;27:847-60.

Moon WJ, Jung SL, Lee JH, et al. Benign and malignant thyroid nodules: US differentiation—multicenter retrospective study. Radiology 2008;247:762-70.

Boey J, Hsu C, Wong J, Ong GB. Fine-needle aspiration versus drill-needle biopsy of thyroid nodules: a controlled clinical trial. Surgery 1982;91:611-5.

Prinz RA, O'Morchoe PJ, Barbato AL, et al. Fine needle aspiration biopsy of thyroid nodules. Ann Surg 1983;198:70-3.

Hundahl SA, Fleming ID, Fremgen AM, Menck HR. A National Cancer Data Base report on 53,856 cases of thyroid carcinoma treated in the U.S., 1985-1995. Cancer 1998;83:2638-48.

Lang BH, Chow SM, Lo CY, et al. Staging systems for papillary thyroid carcinoma: a study of 2 tertiary referral centers. Ann Surg 2007;246:114-21.

Sanders LE, Cady B. Differentiated thyroid cancer: reexamination of risk groups and outcome of treatment. Arch Surg 1998;133:419-25.

Bellantone R, Lombardi CP, Bossola M, et al. Video-assisted vs conventional thyroid lobectomy: a randomized trial. Arch Surg 2002;137:301-4.

Stojadinovic A, Shaha AR, Orlikoff RF, et al. Prospective functional voice assessment in patients undergoing thyroid surgery. Ann Surg 2002;236:823-32.

Wang W, Larson SM, Fazzari M et al. Prognostic value of [18F]fluorodeoxyglucose positron emission tomographic scanning in patients with thyroid cancer. J Clin Endocrinol Metab 2000;85:1107-13.

Palmedo H, Bucerius J, Joe A, et al. Integrated PET/CT in differentiated thyroid cancer: diagnostic accuracy and impact on patient management. J Nucl Med 2006;47:616-24.

UTERINE CANCER

Altekruse SF, Kosary CL, Krapcho M, Neyman N, Aminou R, Waldron W, Ruhl J, Howlader N, Tatalovich Z, Cho H, Mariotto A, Eisner MP, Lewis DR, Cronin K, Chen HS, Feuer EJ, Stinchcomb DG, Edwards BK (eds). SEER Cancer Statistics Review, 1975-2007, National Cancer Institute. Bethesda, MD, http://seer.cancer.gov/csr/1975_2007/, based on November 2009 SEER data submission, posted to the SEER web site, 2010.

Voight LF, Weiss NS. Epidemiology of endometrial cancer. Cancer Treat Res 1989; 49:1-21.

Antunes CM, Strolley PD, Roesenshein NB, et al. Endometrial cancer and estrogen use. Report of a large case-control study. N Eng J Med 1979;300:9-13.

Brinton LA, Berman ML, Mortel R, et al. Reproductive, menstrual, and medical risk factors for endometrial cancer: results from a case-control study. Am J Obstet Gynecol 1992;167:1317-25.

Voight LF, Weiss NS, Chu J, et al. Progestagen supplementation of exogenous oestrogens and risk of endometrial cancer. Lancet 1991;338:274-7.

Pike MC, Peters RK, Cozen W, et al. Estrogen-progestin replacement therapy and endometrial cancer. J Natl Cancer Inst 1997;89:1110-6.

Reeves GK, Pirie K, Beral V, et al. Cancer incidence and mortality in relation to body mass index in the Million Women Study: cohort study. BMJ 2007;335:1134.

Hardiman P, Pillay OC, Atiomo W. Polycystic ovary syndrome and endometrial carcinoma. Lancet 2003;361:1810-2.

Duk JM, Aalders JG, Fleuren GJ, de Bruijn HW. CA 125: a useful marker in endometrial carcinoma. Am J Obstet Gynecol 1986;155:1097-102.

Corpus Uteri. In: Edge SB, Byrd DR, Compton CC, eds. *AJCC Cancer Staging Manual.* 7th ed. New York, NY: Springer, 2010, pp. 403-18.

Benedetti PP, Basile S, Maneschi F, et al. Systematic pelvic lymphadenectomy vs. no lymphadenectomy in early-stage endometrial carcinoma: a randomized clinical trial. J Natl Cancer Inst 2008;100:1707-16.

Kitchener H, Swart AM, Qian Q, et al. Efficacy of systematic pelvic lymphadenectomy in endometrial cancer (MRC ASTEC trial): a randomized study. Lancet 2009;373:125-36.

Zullo F, Palumbo S, Russo T, et al. A prospective randomized comparison between laparoscopic and laparotomic approaches in women with early stage endometrial cancer: focus on the quality of life. Am J Obstet Gynecol 2005;193:1344-52.

Kornblith AB, Huang HQ, Walker JL, et al. Quality of life of patients with endometrial cancer undergoing laparoscopic international federation of gynecology and obstetrics staging compared with laparotomy: a Gynecologic Oncology Group study. J Clin Oncol 2009;27:5337-42.

Aalders J, Abeler V, Kolstad P, Onsrud M. Postoperative external irradiation and prognostic parameters in stage I endometrial carcinoma: clinical and histopathologic study of 540 patients. Obstet Gynecol 1980;56:419-27.

Creutzberg CL, van Putten WL, Koper PC, et al. Surgery and postoperative radiotherapy versus surgery alone for patients with stage-1 endometrial carcinoma: multicentre randomized trial. PORTEC Study Group. Post Operative Radiation Therapy in Endometrial Carcinoma. Lancet 2000;355:1404-11.

Nout RA, Smit VT, Putter H, et al. Vaginal brachytherapy versus pelvic external beam radiotherapy for patients with endometrial cancer of high-intermediate risk (POR-TEC-2): an open-label, non-inferiority, randomised trial. Lancet 2010;375:816-23.

Blake P, Swart AM, Orton J, et al. Adjuvant external beam radiotherapy in the treatment of endometrial cancer (MRC ASTEC and NCIC CTG EN.5 randomized trials): pooled trial results, systematic review, and meta-analysis. Lancet 2009;373:137-46.

Thigpen JT, Brady MF, Homesley HD, et al.: Phase III trial of doxorubicin with or without cisplatin in advanced endometrial carcinoma: a Gynecologic Oncology Group study. J Clin Oncol 2004;22:3902-8.

Randall ME, Filiaci VL, Muss H, et al.: Randomized phase III trial of whole-abdominal irradiation versus doxorubicin and cisplatin chemotherapy in advanced endometrial carcinoma: a Gynecologic Oncology Group Study. J Clin Oncol 2006;24:36-44.

Carey MDS, Gawlik C, Fung-Kee-Fung M, et al. Systematic review of systemic therapy for advanced or recurrent endometrial cancer. Gynecol Oncol 2006;101:158-67.

Homesley HD, Filiaci V, Gibbons SK, et al. A randomized phase III trial in advanced endometrial carcinoma of surgery and volume directed radiation followed by cisplatin and doxorubicin with or without paclitaxel: a Gynecologic Oncology Group study. Gynecol Oncol 2009;112:543-52.